VIDEOENDOSCOPY:
from
VELOPHARYNX
to
LARYNX

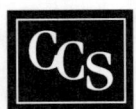

Clinical Competence Series

Series Editor
Robert T. Wertz, Ph.D.

Videoendoscopy: From Velophanyng to Larnyx
Michael P. Karnell, Ph.D

Manual of Voice Treatment: Pediatrics Through Geriatrics
Moya Andrews, Ed.D.

Clinical Manual of Laryngectomy and Head and Neck
Cancer Rehabilitation
Janina K. Casper, Ph.D., and Raymond H. Colton, Ph.D.

Sourcebook for Medical Speech Pathology
Lee Ann C. Golper, Ph.D., CCC-SLP

VIDEOENDOSCOPY:
from
VELOPHARYNX
to
LARYNX

Michael P. Karnell, Ph.D.

The University of Iowa
Department of Otolaryngology-Head and Neck Surgery
Department of Speech Pathology and Audiology

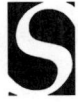

SINGULAR PUBLISHING GROUP, INC.

SAN DIEGO, CALIFORNIA

Singular Publishing Group, Inc.
4284 41st Street
San Diego, California 92105-1197

© 1994 by Singular Publishing Group, Inc.

Typeset in 10/12 Times by ExecuStaff
Printed in the United States of America by McNaughton & Gunn

Library of Congress Cataloging-in-Publication Data

Karnell, Michael P.
  Videoendoscopy : from velopharynx to larynx / Michael P. Karnell.
    p.   cm. — (Clinical competence series)
  Includes bibliographical references and index.
  ISBN 1-879105-97-7
  1. Laryngoscopy.   2. Video endoscopy.   3. Rhinolaryngoscopy.
    [DNLM: 1. Larynx.   2. Laryngoscopy—methods.   3. Pharynx.
  4. Palate, Soft.   5. Video Recording.   WV 505 K18v 1994]
  RF514.K37   1994
  617.5'33059—dc20
  DNLM/DLC
  for Library of Congress   94-12297
                                                                    CIP

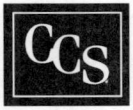

CONTENTS

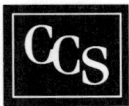

FOREWORD

com · pe· tence (kɔm'pə tə ns) n. The state or quality
of being properly or well qualified; capable.

Clinicians crave competence. They pursue it through education and experience, through emulation and innovation. Some are more successful than others in attaining what they seek. This book by Michael P. Karnell, *Videoendoscopy: From Velopharynx to Larynx,* is one of several in the Singular Clinical Competence Series. Like the others, it is designed to move each of us further along the path that leads to clinical competence. Dr. Karnell describes a tool — videoendoscopy. The use of a tool requires training. Dr. Karnell provides that in the pages that follow. If we master what he tells us, we will increase what we know and improve what we do. His purpose is to create competent clinicians who know the curent body of knowledge about videoendoscopy; have the ability to add continuously to that knowledge; and can apply that knowledge in their appraisal, diagnosis, and treatment. These clinicians will know that no principle, technique, or tool is true or useful until it has been tested; that tests or instruments do not diagnose, and treatments do not treat — clinicians do. Dr. Karnell has developed those traits. His book conveys what makes him competent. Your attention to what he provides indicates your competence and your effort to improve it, because competent clinicians seek competence as much for what it demands as for what it promises.

Robert T. Wertz, Ph.D.
Series Editor

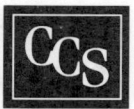

PREFACE

This text communicates a philosophy for including videoendoscopic procedures as part of the Speech Production Assessment Protocol for selected patients. Readers will learn why videoendoscopy is performed, when it should be performed, who should perform it and where, what instrumentation and techniques are useful, what specialized procedures are available and how they are used, how videoendoscopic data are stored and retrieved, and how the data are interpreted. The text draws heavily on photographic excerpts from videoendoscopic and videostroboscopic evaluations to exemplify the issues raised.

Endoscopy is a procedure that traditionally has been limited to the hands of the physician and used for the purposes of identifying disease. Now, most health care providers recognize that endoscopy, when used as a tool for observing the movements of the articulatory and vocal structures involved in speech production, may be used by other health care professionals (e.g., speech pathologists, who have extensive training in understanding and interpreting those movements). An important reason for giving special consideration to endoscopy in this volume is to help clarify this issue so that it may be more appropriately applied to clinical and research applications involving speech in general and resonance and voice in particular.

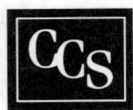

ACKNOWLEDGMENTS

Thanks are extended to Kay Elemetrics Corporation and Olympus Corporation for contributing photographs. Appreciation also to Lucy Hynds Karnell for her artwork. Special thanks to my colleagues Joseph Stemple, Janina Casper, Christy Ludlow, and Hughlett Morris and for their valuable suggestions.

Dedication

To Hughlett Morris and Clyde Willis whose mentoring is in large measure reflected in these pages.

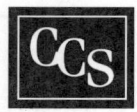

CHAPTER

1

Rationale for Performing Endoscopy

I. WHAT IS ENDOSCOPY?

Endoscopy, generally, is a method for viewing internal body structures. It involves use of an endoscope: a tube containing a system of optical light transmission channels and lenses. Typically, the tube is passed through a natural body opening or a small incision. Internal body structures may be observed by looking through the external side of the tube. Records of endoscopic examinations are possible by coupling photographic, cinegraphic, or, more recently, videographic equipment to the endoscope. The least expensive and most convenient way to record structures within the body currently involves videotape recording of endoscopic images, hence the term videoendoscopy.

1

II. HOW IS ENDOSCOPY APPLIED TO HEALTH CARE?

A. Medical Applications

Endoscopy traditionally has been considered a medical tool and has been used for **both diagnostic and surgical applications.** The nose, throat, bronchi, esophagus, stomach, and intestines are only a few internal body passages that are routinely examined endoscopically. The application of endoscopes to guide joint, sinus, gastric, and ovarian surgery has reduced recovery and rehabilitation time because only very small incisions are necessary.

B. Speech Applications

Endoscopy was popularized as **a tool for the diagnosis and evaluation of speech disorders** by Taub (1966) when he described his oral panendoscope nearly 30 years ago. The oral panendoscope (Figure 1–1) was a rigid device of relatively large diameter making its use in children and small adults difficult. The term *pan*endoscope was adopted, because it was designed to permit rotation of the lens on the distal tip without rotating the entire instrument, allowing the operator to "pan" across structures of interest. A strength of the oral panendoscope was that it could be used to acquire simultaneous audio and moving picture recordings of both the laryngeal and palatopharyngeal structures. Willis and Stutz (1972) described how the panendoscope could be coupled with portable videotape equipment for routine clinical use. A major disadvantage of the panendoscope was that it incorporated a heat producing incandescent light bulb located at the distal tip of the instrument for internal illumination. Consequently, it was necessary to use a heat shield to protect the patient from oral and oropharyngeal burns during use. The heat shield added to the already large diameter of the device making it difficult to tolerate for many patients.

Pigott (1969) described a 3 mm rigid pediatric urethroscope that he applied to visualization of the velopharyngeal mechanism (Figure 1–2). Illumination was provided by a fiberoptic system which eliminated the problems associated with incandescent illumination. Pigott recommended nasal insertion of the scope to avoid interfering with oral articulatory function. At the time of his original report, Pigott advocated the use of a "partially flexible" device in order to make the procedure "less dangerous" for use in

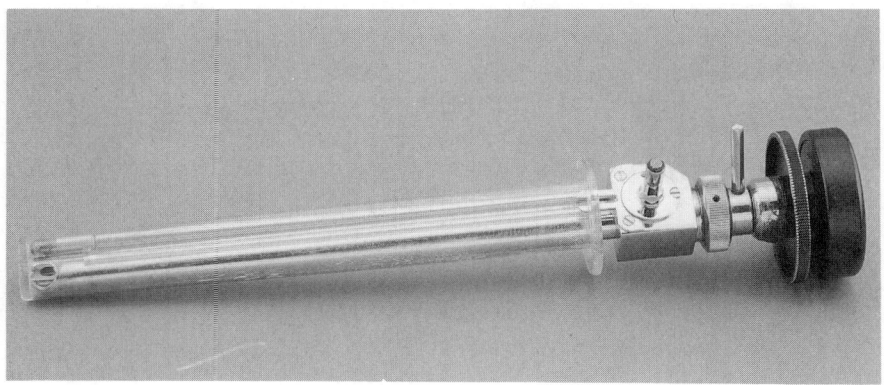

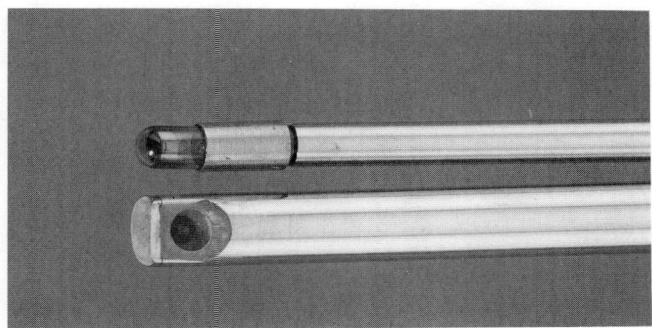

Figure 1–1. The Taub Oral Panendoscope. The insertion tube was encased in a heat shield to protect the patient from the heat generated by the incandescent bulb (**top**). A closeup of the insertion tube without the heat shield is also shown (**bottom**).

small children. However, a few practitioners continue to advocate nasal insertion of rigid endoscopes for evaluation of the velopharyngeal mechanism due to the superior optical characteristics of the rigid endoscopes compared to flexible endoscopes.

Since the early 1970s, substantial advances have occurred in the design of both rigid and flexible endoscopes. Nasal endoscopes have become smaller in diameter, the light transmission characteristics of fiberoptic materials have improved, and fiberoptic light sources have become brighter. In addition, video cameras have become more light sensitive and video tape recorders and monitors have become brighter and sharper. In addition, all of these components have become more affordable. Consequently, the

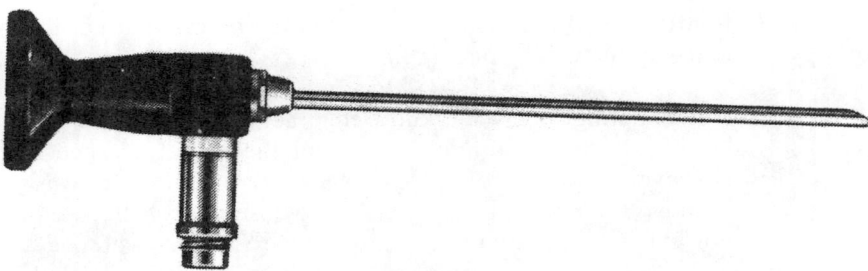

Figure 1–2. The Storz Pigott 3 mm rigid endoscope.

availability and use of endoscopic techniques for evaluation of speech has grown.

III. WHY VIDEOENDOSCOPY?

The motivations for performing videoendoscopy for evaluation of speech and voice are many. Here, we will consider several primary as well as secondary purposes. Primary purposes are those that assist in the initial, **diagnostic** process. Secondary purposes are those that are important for **treatment**.

A. Primary Purposes

It is important from the outset to be clear about the rationale for including endoscopy as a component of the complete evaluation of speech and voice production. There are **three primary purposes for performing endoscopy**:

- To **identify** the physiologic correlates of perceived resonance and voice quality for speech

- To **document** the status of speech anatomy and physiology during speech production

- To **assist** educational and clinical discussion among clinicians, patients, and other interested individuals.

1. **Identifying the physiologic correlates of resonance and voice quality for speech**

It is tempting to assume knowledge about how the oral and laryngeal structures move based on the sound of speech. However, it has become clear that there are multiple ways to move these structures to achieve a desired acoustic result. For example, there are very gifted pipe smokers who speak quite clearly while clenching a pipe between their teeth, effectively eliminating jaw movements. Ventriloquists manage to produce a broad variety of speech sounds while severely limiting lip and jaw movements. It is also clear that individuals with speech disorders can be quite creative in how they move the components of the vocal tract. It is important, therefore, to **obtain objective physiologic information when attempting to understand speech physiology**. Acoustic and perceptual information are important but inadequate when considered alone.

2. **Documenting the status of speech anatomy and physiology during speech production**

It is frequently impossible to capture the complexities of speech movements adequately using verbal descriptions about how those movements appear during speech. Videoendoscopy enables the examiner to record permanently on videotape those movements as viewed through the endoscope. Once this is accomplished, the **view of each speech movement can be reviewed multiple times** by as many professionals as desired so that the most accurate understanding of the events can be achieved, even after the patient has left the clinic.

Another important aspect of the documentation rationale is that it provides **an objective means of identifying the effects of treatment over time**. Multiple video recordings of individual patients can be viewed sequentially in order to demonstrate clearly the success or failure of treatment. This minimizes the risks of failing to identify improvement or falsely assuming improvement based on clinic notes and what can be recalled from previous evaluations.

3. **Assisting educational and clinical discussion among clinicians, patients, and other interested individuals**

For the patient, there is frequently a sense of satisfaction that accompanies the ability to view the structural movements that relate to what they perceive as "hoarse voice" or "nasal speech." In this manner, **videoendoscopy helps remove some of the mystery of their problem**. Review of the video recording with the clinician provides an opportunity for the clinician to point out the source(s) of the problem clearly and educate the patient about the various treatment approaches available. Consequently, patient motivation to follow through with treatment recommendations may improve. The patient and clinician also have an opportunity to absorb and appreciate the implications of the evaluation better compared to when both are occupied by the procedure itself.

Videoendoscopy enables **treatment design** to proceed with a level of confidence that is impossible to achieve when assessment is limited only to the patient's history, what is heard of the patient's speech, and what information may have been passed along by the physician. The video tape record serves as a common source of multidisciplinary diagnostic information from which medical and behavioral management plans may be derived. The videotaped images can be played back multiple times for the referring physicians, students, and other interested health care providers. All can view and discuss the video record without the limitations presented by the patient's presence. This process frequently results in a more accurate and complete diagnosis and treatment plan. When the patient is not present, both health care providers and students may ask questions that might not be appropriate if the patient were present.

B. Secondary Purposes

Secondary purposes of videoendoscopy include:

- Confirmation of medical diagnosis

- Improving patient counseling and motivation

- Providing biofeedback therapy

1. Confirmation of prior diagnosis

It is not uncommon for a medically significant abnormality that was present at the time of an initial medical evaluation to have changed at some later time regardless whether treatment was implemented. It is also not uncommon that the interpretation of physiology by one health care provider can differ from the interpretation of another. Therefore, when a patient is referred for speech or voice therapy due to velopharyngeal insufficiency or a voice disorder, it is always advisable to reexamine the patient to **confirm the presence of the medically diagnosed disorder** prior to beginning behavioral treatment.

An interpretation that differs from that of a health care professional who first evaluated the patient is not correct simply because it is different. Also, there is no question that it is a medical doctor's responsibility to provide the medical diagnosis. The speech-language pathologist who includes videoendoscopy as part of the comprehensive speech/voice evaluation and who sees the problem differently from the patient's primary medical caregiver must decide whether a difference in interpretation is significant enough to warrant a conference with the primary caregiver. For example, a lesion that was reported by the medical doctor as a nodule but appears to the speech-language pathologist more like a polyp may influence the timing and type of behavioral management the speech-language pathologist deems appropriate. The video record frequently serves to help both parties agree on the nature of the problem and the appropriate management options. However, if the difference is one of semantics rather than substance and will not influence the manner in which the patient is to be treated, simple notation of observations in the patient's record will usually be sufficient. Above all, it must be remembered by all involved that the **videoendoscopic study is performed to benefit the patient**; not to encourage clinical rivalry or turf disputes.

2. Improving patient counseling and motivation

As stated previously, it is easier for a patient to grasp the nature of his or her problem when reviewing the videotape record of the videoendoscopic examination. However, it warrants special emphasis that such review may have the **added benefit of increasing patient motivation** to participate in and follow through with treatment recommendations. This is particularly important where speech and voice therapy are concerned. Patients are frequently disappointed when the treatment for their problem involves more investment on their part than taking medication or even undergoing a surgical procedure. Therapy requires from the patient a major committment of time, energy, and money. Therefore, the video record is useful to show the patient visually how therapy would help, why other methods of treatment are not indicated, and what the ultimate consequences of noncompliance with treatment might be.

3. Providing biofeedback therapy

Biofeedback has been shown to be **a useful approach to certain problems in select patients**. Stated simply, biofeedback is a means by which an individual learns to alter a biological or behavioral process by monitoring the process. Such monitoring may be visual, auditory, or tactile, but regardless of medium, the effect of monitoring is to give individuals some information about the state of the biological process they wish to change and the effects of their efforts to alter that state. For example, some patients are able to reduce heart rate while monitoring their heart rate via audible feedback.

The use of videoendoscopy as a biofeedback channel to alter velopharyngeal closure for speech (Siegel-Sadewitz & Shprintzen, 1982) and laryngeal movements (Bastian & Nagorsky, 1987) has been suggested. However, there is no convincing evidence to support its clinical use as a biofeedback device on a routine basis at this time. Some patients appear able to make adjustments in velar physiology while monitoring a video image of their velopharyngeal mechanism. More research is needed to determine how generalizable biofeedback may be to other patients and other speaking environments.

A potential problem with biofeedback applications of videoendoscopy is that they require **prolonged placement of the endoscope**. Such prolonged placement can have secondary effects. For example, patient discomfort and copious mucus production, that limit the effectiveness of the technique. Additional study is needed of this very interesting and compelling application of videoendoscopy.

IV. WHO SHOULD DO VIDEOENDOSCOPY?

In general, the best person to perform the videoendoscopic evaluation of speech physiology is the person who is most competent to obtain accurate information about physiologic function without placing the patient at risk. Note that this makes no assumptions about academic degree. Currently, there is no specific course of study that one may pursue to become a skilled endoscopist. Those who use the procedure, both physician and nonphysician, learn to do so during the processes of managing patients clinically or performing research.

A. Medical Personnel

There were several reasons why endoscopy was traditionally limited to physicians. As stated above, the initial applications for endoscopy were to identify disease processes or assist surgery. Another reason for limiting the procedure to physicians' hands related to the internal placement of the endoscope. It has been assumed that there were significant risks associated with placement of the nasal endoscope and nasal application of topical anesthetics. such as nasal irritation and bleeding, fainting, and laryngospasm that could jeopardize patient safety. It has always been, and remains now, the physician's responsibility to treat whatever medical complications might arise from the procedure.

It has become clear that, although there are important risks involved with some forms of endoscopy, those **risks can be minimized** by controlling the environment in which the procedure is performed and providing adequate training for the endoscopist. The issue of risks will be considered in more detail later in this volume.

When the purpose of the endoscopic examination is to evaluate speech and voice, the effectiveness of the procedure may be limited if the procedure is restricted to the physician. Medical students frequently receive limited education regarding speech and voice production. Indeed, the discipline of speech-language pathology evolved, in part, due to the recognition of physicians, psychologists, educators, and linguists that there was need for professionals who have specialized knowledge about speech production and who are qualified to apply that knowledge clinically (Moeller. 1976). Fully trained, certified, licensed speech-language pathologists provide the expertise necessary to make endoscopic evaluation of speech and voice appropriate and meaningful.

B. Nonmedical personnel

Nonmedical personel began to become involved in videoendo-scopy as more behavioral, nonmedical applications for video-endoscopy were identified. For example, a major task of speech-language pathologists involved in assessing the speech of individuals with cleft palate or craniofacial abnormalities has been to determine the **adequacy of velopharyngeal closure** for speech production. In an effort to be more objective, speech pa-thologists enhanced their clinical judgments of perceived oral/nasal resonance balance with instrumentation. Included were analyses of speech acoustics and aerodyamics and observation of videofluorographic images of speech physiology. Videoendoscopic imaging of speech physiology was a natural extension of these attempts to expand and improve speech and voice evaluations.

Speech-language pathologists have been performing videoen-doscopy as part of the clinical and research process for more than 20 years beginning prior to the advent of flexible fiberoptic endoscopes. The rigid oral endoscopes first applied to speech and voice evaluation (Taub, 1966) were easily adapted by speech-language pathologists who were already including in their clini-cal regimen indirect mirror examination of velopharyngeal and la-ryngeal structures (Willis & Stutz, 1972). When flexible fiberoptic endoscopes became available, speech-language pathologists who had been using oral endoscopy began using nasal endoscopy as well, with the support and assistance of their medical colleagues.

Several issues regarding risks have emerged as more speech-language pathologists have become involved in endoscopic pro-cedures. The first of these has to do with **differences between a medical examination and a speech examination**. As stated previously, the purpose of the medical examination is the identi-fication of disease. During these examinations, the patient is ex-pected to tolerate discomfort, and the physician is expected to be thorough in the search for the problem. The purpose of the speech examination is to evaluate speech and voice production. Patient comfort and cooperation are paramount if accurate and valid in-formation about speech behavior is desired. An agitated, uncom-fortable patient is not likely to provide the examiner with a sample of speech representative of her or his typical conversational speech. Thus, endoscopy in a speech evaluation must be performed with care and with special attention to patient cooperation and comfort. The chances of patient injury under these circumstances is reduced relative to the medical evaluation.

Another issue related to risks involves the use of **anesthetics**. Oral videoendoscopy usually does not require use of anesthetics and, therefore, has no associated risks. However, most clinicians who perform nasal endoscopy prefer to employ topical anesthetics to reduce patient sensitivity to insertion of the nasal endoscope. Flexible endoscopes used for nasal videoendoscopy have become smaller as fiberoptic technology has advanced. As the endoscopes have become smaller, so too has the need for anesthesia. In fact, the discomfort associated with the application of anesthesia is frequently more a source of patient complaint than the discomfort associated with scope placement. Watterson (1992) has stated that he routinely performs nasal endoscopy without the use of topical anesthetics, although he acknowledges limiting his application to adult patients.

The main risk of anesthetics is not **overdose**. Typically, the amount of anesthesia necessary to achieve the desired reduction in nasal sensitivity for a given individual is quite small and, as will be illustrated later, well below the amount that would place the typical patient at risk of overdose. The primary risk to patient safety associated with topical anesthetics is **allergic reaction**. Such reactions can result in rapid swelling of tissue that can inhibit the patient's ability to breathe. Precautions must be taken, therefore, in preparation for the rare patient who suffers an allergic reaction. An adequate precaution is to perform nasal videoendoscopy only in medical clinics where medical contingency plans are in place to handle clinical emergencies.

Speech-language pathologists receive special training in the anatomy and physiology of normal speech production and in the behavioral manipulation of disordered speech. This training is directly applicable to eliciting patient cooperation during the videoendoscopic examination, determining which speech and voice behaviors to observe during the videoendoscopic examination, and directing patient speech and voice behavior in order to observe the anatomical and physiologic correlates of speech and voice production. The best qualified professional to perform the videoendoscopic evaluation of speech and voice production is clearly the speech-language pathologist.

The **benefits** of including the endoscopic examination as part of the speech physiology examination far outweigh the potential **risks**. Recognition that this procedure is used by nonmedically trained health care providers such as speech-language pathologists has grown. A strong partnership between the speech-language pathologist, the medical doctor, and the facility in which video-endoscopy is performed provides the most effective and safest environment for the videoendoscopic evaluation of speech and voice production.

V. SPECIALIZED TRAINING FOR VIDEOENDOSCOPY

There has been no formal course of study available for medical or nonmedical professionals who perform videoendoscopy. Medical students and residents typically learn the procedure informally by observing attending physicians or more senior students handle the in-struments. Similarly, speech-language pathologists learn the procedure from **informal observation**. Although this may not be the optimal way to learn how to perform endoscopy, it is clear that informal train-ing has not impaired most interested clinicians from acquiring the skill and applying it effectively.

Beyond learning the technical details of performing the procedure, there is need for training about **interpretation**. There have been more structured, formal educational experiences regarding interpretation. These have typically taken the form of short courses, seminars, and workshops offered during regional or national meetings for medical doctors, speech-language pathologists, or both.

The need for formal training in videoendoscopic procedures and in-terpretation requires discussion. It seems logical that training should include specific periods of structured lecture, observation, practice, and discussion. Lecture is needed to clarify the purpose of the pro-cedure and to provide a conceptual framework for later observation and practice. It is also an important method for teaching interpreta-tion of videoendoscopic data. Observation and practice are required to provide opportunities for mastering the technical details and fine motor skills necessary to become competent to perform the proce-dure clinically. These experiences could be provided during a work-shop over the course of a few days. However, **true mastery and competence** should not be expected until considerably more clini-cal experience with the procedure has been obtained over a period of months or, perhaps, years.

It is not clear how much experience is needed or whether there should be a structured period of supervised internship beyond the initial training period. Ultimately, initial training for videoendoscopy should be incorporated into **clinical training programs** for physicians and speech-language pathologists. Workshops should be made available for those who wish to acquire the skill or expand their range of video-endoscopic competence after graduation from clinical training.

VI. WHERE TO DO VIDEOENDOSCOPY

The most suitable location to perform videoendoscopy depends on whether the endoscope is to be inserted nasally or orally and whether anesthetics are used.

A. Oral Endoscopy Without Anesthetics

Oral endoscopy performed for the purpose of evaluation of speech does not require anesthetics and can be performed in any clinical environment prepared to support the procedure. Support means having the necessary equipment, material, and expertise to perform the procedure and to clean and disinfect the endoscope thoroughly. It is not necessary, therefore, to perform oral endoscopy in a medical setting.

B. Nasal or Oral Endoscopy With Anesthetics

When videoendoscopy requires anesthesia and/or nasal insertion, the procedure should be limited to an environment where there is **full medical support**. Thus, if the patient suffers a reaction that requires immediate medical attention, that attention can be made available within seconds. A medical clinic with emergency procedures clearly documented and available is necessary. Whoever performs the procedure must be familiar with emergency procedures and certified in **cardiopulmonary resuscitation** given the possibility of respiratory distress. However, the presence of a physician during every videoendoscopic speech and voice evaluation is excessive and unnecessary.

VII. FOR WHOM IS VIDEOENDOSCOPY APPROPRIATE?

Videoendoscopy is a preferred diagnostic procedure for patients who have **velopharyngeal** and/or **laryngeal disorders** that affect **speech**

production. This includes patients who are hypernasal, patients who exhibit audible nasal emission of air during speech production, and patients who are dysphonic or who are complaining about limited vocal ability. There is also a role for videoendoscopy in the assessment of swallowing.

When used for the assessment of speech, videoendoscopy requires a **cooperative, speaking patient**. Patients who are noncooperative or who are nonverbal due to central nervous system disorder, hearing impairment, or other anomaly are not appropriate candidates. Also, patients who are physically too small or immature to tolerate the procedure are not good candidates. However, the diameter of the endoscopic insertion tube and the skill of the endoscopist help determine how large and cooperative a patient may be before a successful examination can be expected. Children as young as 3 years of age have tolerated nasal endoscopy when a small endoscope (3 mm outside diameter or less), adequate patient preparation, and coaching are used. The details of preparation and coaching will be discussed later.

Patients who have a **history of significant health problems** require special consideration before performing videoendoscopy. The policies of health care facilities vary regarding how these patients should be managed. Patients with compromised immune systems, heart valve problems, or allergies to anesthetics require approval from a physician before nasal videoendoscopy is performed or before anesthetics are administered. When the procedure is performed with these patients, it should be limited to health care settings that can provide the necessary support if a patient experiences difficulty. Typically, many of these patients have received endoscopic examinations prior to being referred for a speech and voice videoendoscopic examination by their physician. Precautions are usually communicated by the referring physician, the patient, or both. The endoscopist should always ask the patient whether he or she has had **endoscopy** and whether there were any **associated difficulties**.

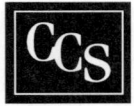

CHAPTER

2

Anatomy and Physiology

Performing flexible nasal or rigid oral videoendoscopy requires special knowledge and skills. Nasal and pharyngeal anatomy and physiology vary among patients. **Clear understanding of both normal and abnormal anatomy and physiology is essential** for the endoscopist.

I. THE NASAL PASSAGES

The nasal passages are complex, quasi-horizontal chambers in the upright patient. They extend from the nares anteriorly to the velopharyngeal port posteriorly and from the floor of the palate inferiorly to the base of the skull superiorly. The left and right nasal passages are separated by the nasal septum. For our purposes, the anterior, middle, and posterior nasal structures will be considered separately.

15

A. Anterior Nasal Structures

The anterior support structure of the **nose** and **septum** (Figure 2–1) includes the **nasal bones** and associated cartilaginous structures that are covered with mucous membrane internally. Muscle and an overlying layer of dermis cover the external surfaces. The nasal bones articulate rostrally with the frontal bone and extend downward and forward to support the upper one third of the nose. The **nasal cartilages** include the greater alar cartilages which join at the midline to form the tip of the external nose and the lateral nasal cartilages which form the anterior bridge of the nose. The lesser alar cartilages support the structure of the lateral aspect of the nasal ala. Proximal to the nasal cartilages are the bilateral nasal bones which complete the nasal framework.

The **septal cartilage** forms at the proximal union of the left and right greater alar and lateral nasal cartilages and extends posteriorly to form the **anterior nasal septum**. It communicates posteriorly with the perpendicular plate of the ethmoid bone and inferiorly with the premaxilla and maxilla. At the nostrils, the septal cartilage supports the midline nasal columella.

The anterior nose has only **one muscle of endoscopic interest**. The levator labii alaeque nasi originates from the lateral nasal cartilages and courses downward and laterally to insert into the orbicularis oris muscles of the upper lip. When contracted, the

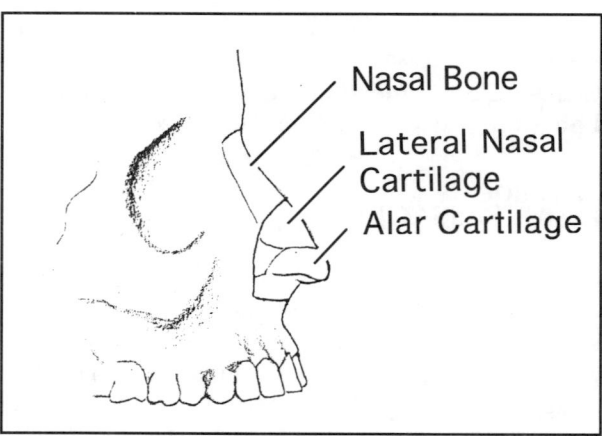

Figure 2–1. The supporting structure of the anterior nose.

muscle assists upper lip elevation. It can also wrinkle the skin overlying the cartilaginous anterior nasal structures, resulting in the familiar facial expression associated with displeasure.

B. Middle Nasal Structure

The supporting structures of the middle nasal passages (Figure 2–2) are primarily bone and include the palate, the posterior nasal septum, and the nasal turbinates.

1. Palate

The anterior bony palate is made up of the paired bones of the **premaxilla**. Posterior to the premaxilla are the paired bones of the **maxilla** which make up the primary bulk of the palate. Further posterior to the maxillary bones are the paired **palatine bones** which form the posterior border of the bony palate.

2. Posterior Nasal Septum

The perpendicular plate of the **ethmoid bone** provides bony structure for the most superior portion of the nasal septum proximal and superior to the cartilaginous framework provided by the septal cartilage described previously. The largest area of the bony septum is made up of the unpaired, midline, vertical **vomer bone** which extends along the

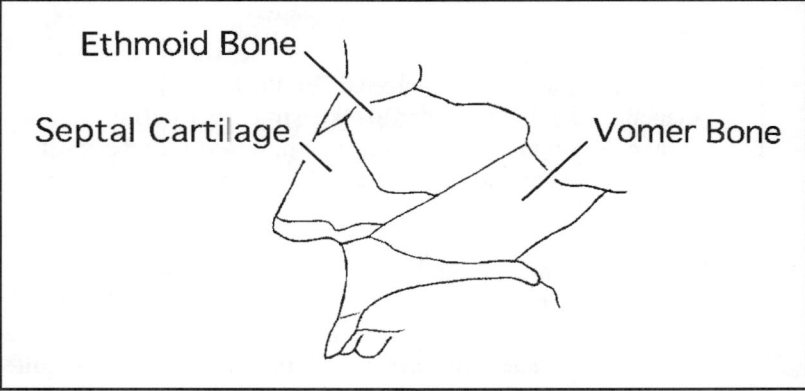

Figure 2–2. The supporting structure of the middle nasal passages.

entire floor of the nasal cavity where it is anchored to the maxillae and palatine bones. It articulates anteriorly with the cartilaginous nasal septum. Superiorly, the vomer articulates with the perpendicular plate of the **ethmoid** and rostrum of the **sphenoid bone**. The posterior edge of the vomer is free, permitting posterior communication of the left and right nasal passages as they extend to the nasopharynx beyond the posterior openings of the nasal cavities called the **nasal choanae**. The nasal septum is of special endoscopic interest because it forms the medial borders of the inferior and middle **nasal meati** through which a nasal endoscope may be passed.

Although the surfaces of the septum are frequently smooth and straight, it is neither uncommon nor necessarily abnormal for bony irregularities to extend from the vomer into the middle or inferior nasal meati. These irregularities make the nasal meati somewhat tortuous and may **complicate insertion of a nasal endoscope**. It is also not uncommon in normal individuals for the entire **nasal septum to be deviated** laterally from its midline location. Septal deviation is almost always apparent in the unilateral **cleft palate** population, since the inferior attachment of the vomer is displaced laterally as the cleft extends through the maxillary and palatine bones. In some individuals the anterior vomer is displaced laterally toward one side while the posterior vomer is displaced laterally toward the opposite side, creating constrictions in both nasal cavities.

3. Nasal Turbinates (conchae) and Meati

The nasal turbinates (also know as the shell-shaped nasal conchae) are of special interest for those involved in nasal videoendoscopy. These scroll-like structures define the two passages through which the endoscope insertion tube must be passed for visualization of the velar, pharyngeal, and laryngeal structures.

The superior and middle nasal turbinates project inferiorly from the medial surfaces of the ethmoid labyrinths which make up the lateral walls of the uppermost portions of the nasal cavities. The **superior nasal turbinate** is usually quite small and difficult to visualize endoscopically because it is positioned above and posterior to the middle turbinate. The

middle turbinate is of special endoscopic interest because it defines the upper border of the **middle nasal meatus**— one of the two major routes for nasal endoscope insertion.

The **inferior nasal turbinates** are bones that form the lateral walls of the nasal cavity inferior to the ethmoid labyrinths with which they communicate superiorly. They are attached inferiorly and laterally along the nasal surface of the maxillae and palatine bones. The body of the inferior turbinate extends from its bony attachments into the lumen of the inferior nasal cavity to form a scroll-like configuration similar to the superior and middle turbinates. It is the largest of the three turbinates and **the most important to identify endoscopically**, as it defines the inferior border of the middle nasal meatus and the superior border of the inferior nasal meatus. The anterior-most portion of the inferior nasal turbinate is usually the first structure observed endoscopically after the endoscope clears the hairs surrounding the anterior nasal vestibule.

The inferior nasal meatus is usually larger in area than the middle meatus. It is, therefore, usually **easier to achieve a successful nasal endoscope insertion through the inferior nasal meatus**. The middle meatus is usually large enough to accomodate a flexible nasal endoscope insertion tube in most men and many women. The lumen of the middle meatus in some women and most children may accommodate only small diameter, pediatric, flexible endoscopes (< 3 mm diameter). The nasal meati may be partially or completely blocked due to nasal turbinate **hypertrophy** (abnormally large nasal turbinates), **septal deviation** or **bone spurs**, or **edema** of the mucous membrane covering the nasal passages.

4. Posterior Nasal Structures—The Nasopharynx

The superior and lateral bony structure of the posterior nasal cavity, or nasopharynx, is made up of the **rostrum** and **medial pterygoid lamina** of the **sphenoid bone** respectively. The superior structure is completed as the dorsal surface of the sphenoid communicates with the basilar portion of the occipital bone anterior to the foramen magnum. When present, the **adenoid tissue** can be visualized via nasal videoendoscopy along these surfaces of the posterior-superior nasopharynx. The posterior wall of the nasopharynx is supported by the body of the atlas, the first cervical vertebra, and the pharyngeal aponeurosis.

The floor of the anterior nasopharynx consists of the **soft palate or velum**. There is no bony support posterior to the palatine bones. The posterior border of the velum is free and defines the anterior border of the velopharyngeal port (Figure 2–3). The **velopharyngeal port** is further defined laterally by the superior constrictor and salpingopharyngeus muscles. It is defined posteriorly by the posterior pharyngeal wall including the pharyngeal aponeurosis and superior constrictor muscle overlying the cervical vertebral column.

II. VELOPHARYNX

The velopharyngeal mechanism **valves the opening between the oral and nasal cavities**. This opening, called the velopharyngeal port, must be adequately valved during oral speech production to prevent **hypernasal resonance** and during swallowing to prevent nasal reflux. It is significant in individuals with congenital **cleft palate** because the function of the mechanism is directly affected by the

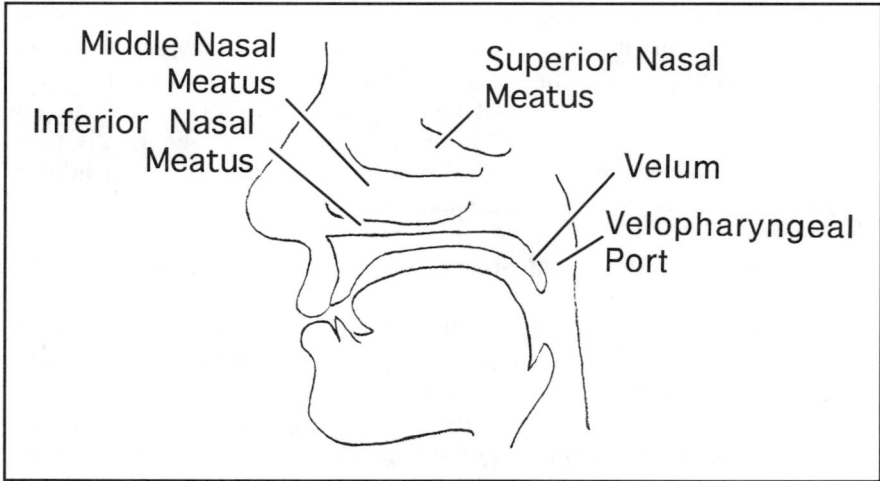

Figure 2–3. The velum (soft palate) occupies the floor of the posterior nasal passage. Also shown are the inferior, middle, and superior nasal meati.

presence of the palatal cleft. Although its function may appear relatively simple and straightforward, velopharyngeal anatomy and physiology are quite complex.

A. Velum

The velum, or soft palate, is made up of **muscle**, the **palatal aponeurosis**, a substantial amount of connective and glandular tissue, and overlying **mucous membrane**. The majority of the palatal bulk consists of the **bilateral levator veli palatini muscles**, each of which arises from the petrous portion of the ipsilateral temporal bone. They extend inferiorly, medially, and anteriorly into the palate where they interdigitate with one another. Levator is secured anteriorly to the ipsilateral palatine bone via the palatal aponeurosis, the tendonous fan-like extension of the **tensor veli palatini** muscle. Each tensor muscle arises near the base of the medial pterygid lamina of the ipsilateral sphenoid and descends to form a tendon which winds around the hamulus, the most inferior process of the medial pterygoid lamina of the sphenoid bone. The tendon then fans out to form the palatal aponeurosis which gives tendonous support to the soft palatal structure and attaches the velum to the palatine bones. Contraction of the levator muscles elevates the velum, whereas contraction of tensor muscles tenses and lowers the palatal aponeurosis. The primary function of each tensor is to open the ipsilateral eustachian tube so that middle ear air pressure may be equalized with atmospheric air pressure.

The **musculus uvulae** is a midline muscle which arises from the palatal aponeurosis. It extends over the fibers of levator and inserts into the uvula, the midline extension of the soft palate. It adds bulk to the palatal midline and upon contraction shortens and lifts the soft palate.

The **palatoglossus muscles** are important muscles of the palate as well as the tongue. Each arises from the oral surface of the palatal aponeurosis and extends downward, forward, and laterally, to insert into the sides of the tongue dorsum. The palatoglossus muscles are contained within the anterior facial arches. Contraction of the palatoglossus muscles lowers the palate.

The **palatopharyngeus muscles** arise from the soft palate posterior to the palatoglossus muscle. A small group of palatopharyngeus fibers may arise from the hamulus and cartilaginous eustachian tube. These fibers are called the **salpingopharyngeus** and make up a bulge known as the **salpingopharyngeal fold** which is visible along the lateral walls of the velopharyngeal port. The fibers of the **palatopharyngeus** are divided by levator as they course downward and laterally. They converge lateral to the levator to form the posterior faucial pillar and then insert inferiorly into the lateral walls of the pharynx. Some fibers also insert into the superior horn of the thyroid cartilage. Contraction of palatopharyngeus may serve to lower the palate, narrow the oral-pharyngeal isthmus (the space between the two posterior facial arches), or elevate the larynx. It is most active during deglutition when it serves to guide the bolus from the oral cavity into the pharynx.

B. Lateral Pharyngeal Walls

At the level of the nasopharynx, the lateral walls of the velopharyngeal port are defined by the **superior constrictor muscles** and the **salpingopharyngeal folds** (Figure 2–4). Visible endoscopically in the nasopharynx lateral to the velum is the torus tubarius, a semicircular bulge of mucous membrane surrounding the nasal opening, or ostium, of the eustachian tube. The posterior border of this bulge overlays the salpingopharyngeal fold containing the salpingopharyngeal muscle.

C. Posterior Pharyngeal Walls

The posterior pharyngeal wall at the level of the nasopharynx includes the **pharyngeal aponeurosis** and **superior pharyngeal constrictor muscles** overlying the cervical vertebral column. Contraction of the upper fibers of the superior constrictor muscle elevates a narrow band of mucous membrane extending laterally along the width of the posterior pharyngeal wall. When present, this elevated tissue is called "**Passavant's ridge**."

III. OROPHARYNX

The **oropharynx is the portion of the pharynx roughly at the level of the oral cavity** (Figure 2–5). It is defined superiorly by the

velopharyngeal port and inferiorly by the superior surface of the **epiglottis**.

A. Anterior Structures

1. Posterior Tongue

Just inferior to the velopharyngeal port is the posterior tongue or tongue dorsum. Viewed endoscopically from above, it appears rather coarse due to the lymph and mucous glands it contains. These make up what is known as the **lingual tonsils**.

2. Valecula

Posterior to the tongue dorsum are depressions known as the valeculae. They are bordered posteriorly by the lingual

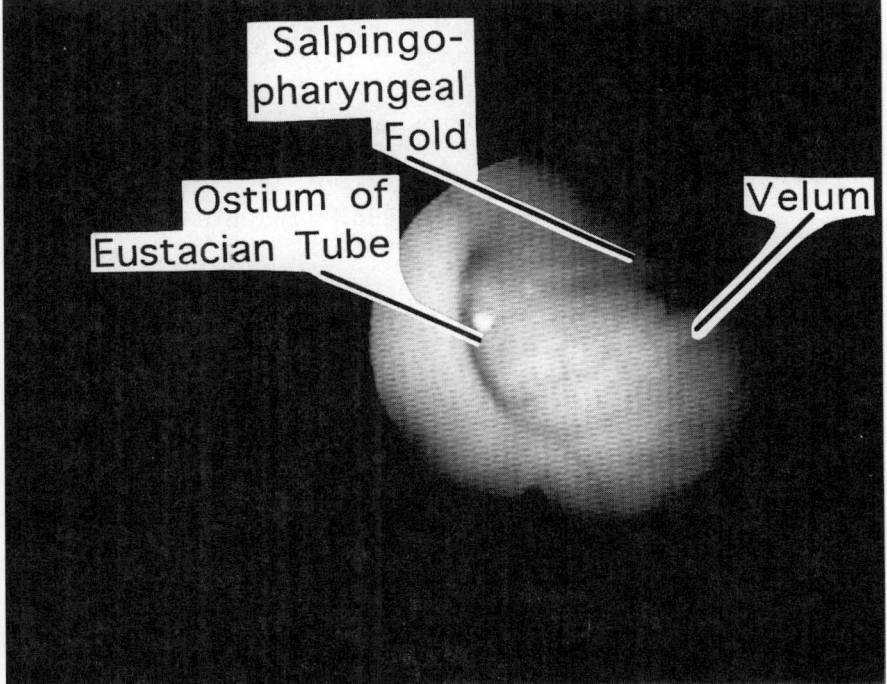

Figure 2–4. Endoscopic view from the right inferior meatus of the right Eustachian tube ostium, salpingopharyngeal fold, and velum.

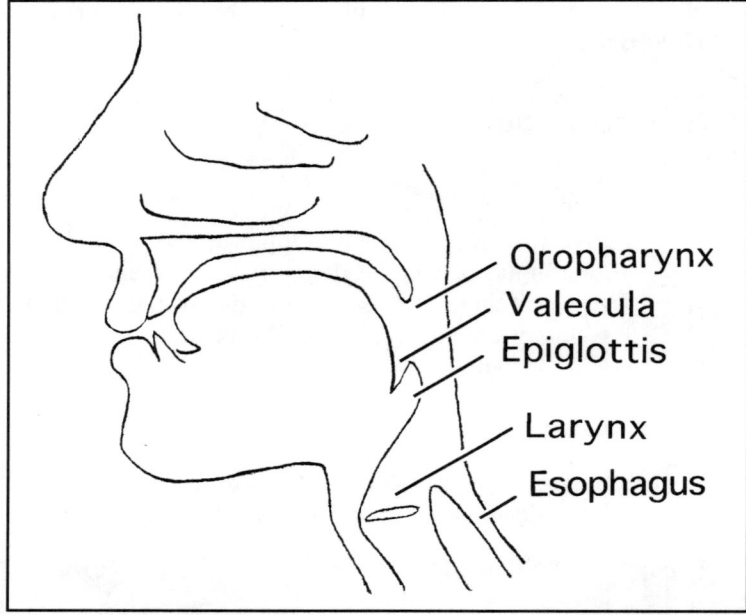

Figure 2–5. The oropharynx including the valecula, or space between the epiglottis and tongue dorsum. The bulk of the epiglottis and larynx are inferior to the oropharynx.

surface of the **superior epiglottis** and divided medially by the **glosso-epiglottic fold**.

B. Lateral and Posterior Pharyngeal Walls

The lateral and posterior pharyngeal walls at the level of the oropharynx contain fibers of the **superior constrictor muscles**. The superior constrictor has a broad and complex origin extending from the medial pterygoid plate superiorly along the pterygomandibular raphe to the sides of the tongue inferiorly. It courses downward and laterally to insert into the median pharyngeal raphe. The posterior wall, at the level of the oropharynx, is supported by the cervical vertebral column.

IV. HYPOPHARYNX

A. Larynx

Immediately inferior to the oropharynx is the hypopharynx which contains the supraglottic structure of the larynx (Figure 2–6).

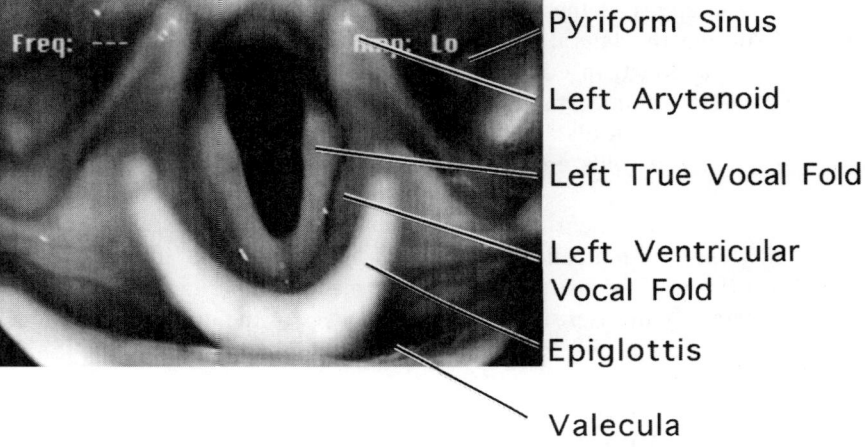

Pyriform Sinus

Left Arytenoid

Left True Vocal Fold

Left Ventricular Vocal Fold

Epiglottis

Valecula

Figure 2–6. An endoscopic view from the oropharynx permits visualization of the pyriform sinuses, arytenoids, true vocal folds, ventricular folds, epiglottis, and valecula.

Endoscopically, the first laryngeal structure encountered is the epiglottis, a broad, curved, cartilaginous structure which narrows inferiorly to its connection with the thyroid cartilage via the thy-roepiglottic ligament. The epiglottis defines the posterior surface of the **valeculae** anteriorly and the entrance to the interior larynx, known as the **laryngeal vestibule**, posteriorly. At the base of the epiglottis, a small bulge called the petiolus is frequently observed.

Extending from the lateral edges of the superior surface of the epiglottis inferiorly and laterally are the **aryepiglottic folds**. These form the lateral sides of the **laryngeal vestibule** and contain some fibers of the oblique arytenoid muscles which may assist epiglottic inversion during deglutition. The aryepiglottic folds communicate with the superior process of the **arytenoid cartilages**. The arytenoid cartilages appear at the base of the aryepiglottic folds as two relatively large, rounded structures. Extending between the arytenoids posteriorly and the base of the epiglottis anteriorly are the **true vocal folds** and, just superior and lateral to the true vocal folds, are the **ventricular vocal folds**. The true vocal folds are visible endoscopically as two smooth, straight bands of pearly white tissue in a V-shaped configuration. The area at the convergence of the two vocal folds is called the **anterior commissure**. The space between the vocal folds at the arytenoid cartilages is the **posterior commissure**.

The edges of the true vocal folds appear relatively sharp as they define the lateral margins of the **glottis**, the space between the vocal folds. In contrast, the ventricular vocal folds appear as bilateral rounded mounds of pink tissue lateral and superior to the true vocal folds. The depressions between the true and ventricular vocal folds are called the **laryngeal ventricles**.

Each true vocal fold contains a band of muscle, the thyroarytenoid, often called the **vocalis**, arising from the angle of the thyroid cartilage anteriorly. These muscles course posteriorly and laterally to insert into the vocal process of the arytenoid cartilages. Proximal to the vocalis muscle are the three layers of the **lamina propria**. The deepest layer is the most stiff of the three and consists of collaginous fibers. The intermediate layer consists of elastic fibers, and the superficial layer consists of a loose, soft, gelatinous matrix. The intermediate and deep layers of the lamina propria make up the vocal ligament. The surface of the vocal folds is covered with squamous epithelium. This complex layered structure of the vocal fold edges is considered **critical for normal vibratory function** (Hirano, 1984).

B. Pyriform Sinus

The most inferior surfaces of the hypopharynx are lateral to the arytenoid cartilages and medial to the lamina of the thyroid cartilage. These bilateral depressions are called the pyriform sinuses.

C. Cricopharyngeus

Immediately posterior to the arytenoid cartilages is a shallow crease. This area is the superior edge of the **esophagus**. It is encircled by the cricopharyngeus muscle which remains in tonic contraction except during deglutition. In some patients, **gastroesophageal (GE) reflux** can be observed emerging from this area. GE reflux may be a serious condition if gastric acids fall onto the laryngeal or subglottic spaces.

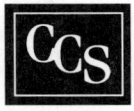

CHAPTER

3

Instrumentation

The successful performance of videoendoscopy requires specialized knowledge of the equipment involved. In this section, instrumentation used for both nasal and oral videoendoscopy will be described. Some technical expertise is needed to manage the equipment involved in performing videoendoscopy. The endoscopist must know about the various endoscopes, cameras, lenses, videotape recorders, and microphones that are needed.

I. ENDOSCOPES

Two types of endoscopes are used for videoendoscopy: flexible and rigid. **Flexible scopes** are designed for **nasal insertion**. The flexible nature of these scopes promotes patient comfort in spite of the sometimes tortuous path of the nasal lumen. **Rigid scopes** are most frequently used for **oral insertion**, although some small diameter scopes have been advocated for nasal insertion also. Although nasal insertion of rigid scopes can provide excellent images in some patients, the relative benefit compared to nasal insertion of flexible scopes is insufficient, given the increased likelihood of patient discomfort and potential for nasal trauma. In general, the type of endoscope selected depends on the purpose for which it is to be used, the physical characteristics of the patient, and the preferences of the endoscopist.

All endoscopes used in videoendoscopy have several components in common; a **viewing lens**, an **insertion tube** with lenses, and a **fiberoptic cable** for light transmission from a light source (Figure 3–1). Light from the light source is transmitted through the fiberoptic cable to the insertion tube where it is then passed along a channel to a light emitting lens at the tip.

The insertion tube is designed for light transmission in two directions. First, it transmits light from the fiberoptic light cable to a light emitting lens on the distal end of the insertion tube. The light emitting lens focuses illumination on the area in front of the lens. If some of the light is reflected back to the tip, that light is directed via a light receiving lens back into the insertion tube and through another channel where it is transmitted to the viewing lens located in the eye-

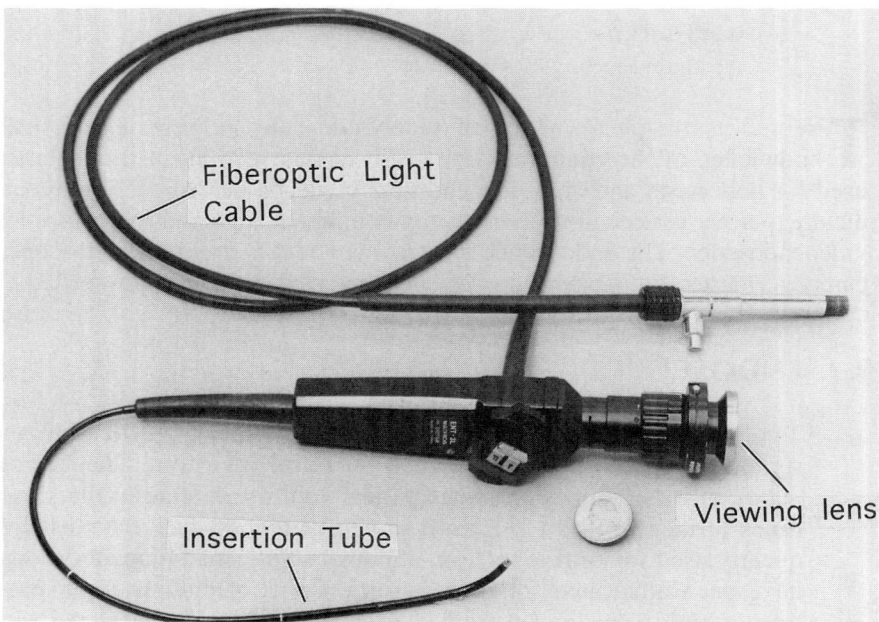

Figure 3–1. Common components of all endoscopes include a viewing lens, insertion tube, and fiberoptic light cable.

piece. The examiner's eye or a video camera positioned at the eyepiece can then view the illuminated structures in front of the insertion tube lens system.

A. Rigid Endoscopes

Rigid endoscopes are those with rigid, metal insertion tubes through which light is transmitted via air-filled channels. Light is transmitted through the insertion tube and from lens to lens in a manner similar to that found in photographic cameras. The lenses on the tip may be arranged at a variety of angles relative to the long axis of the insertion tube. For speech and voice evaluation, rigid scopes with either a **90° or 70° lens angle** are most commonly used. The diameter of rigid scopes varies, again, depending on their intended use.

Rigid scopes have been used for both nasal and oral endoscopy. Nasal insertion of a small diameter (< 3 mm) rigid endoscope is complex because of the frequently tortuous configuration of the nasal passages and the inability of rigid scopes to provide a forward looking view during insertion. Consequently, their use in nasal endoscopy has become rare, particularly as the quality of flexible endoscopes has improved.

Rigid endoscopes are **most useful for oral insertion**. The rigid insertion tube is critical for oral insertion so that the endoscopist can control the placement of the lens for viewing the larynx or velopharynx in the face of interference from tongue movements. Scopes designed for oral use usually have larger (< 3 mm) diameter insertion tubes than nasal scopes allowing for greater light transmitting capacity and, therefore, brighter, clearer images.

For example, if oral endoscopy is performed to evaluate **velopharyngeal function**, a small diameter rigid scope such as the Storz-Pigott Nasopharyngoscope (model 5925C) is useful (shown previously in Figure 1–2). This scope has a 4.2 mm maximum outside diameter and a 70° viewing angle. It is useful for velopharyngeal studies because its relatively small outside diameter makes it easy to achieve complete bilabial closure around the scope during production of [pa] and [ba] syllables. This scope requires a relatively bright light source because the light transmission channel is relatively small.

Laryngeal evaluations performed via oral endoscopy require a larger diameter rigid endoscope like the Nakamichi 70°, the Wolfe 90°, or the Storz 90° models (Figure 3–2). The larger light transmission capabilities of these scopes ensure a sufficiently bright image even during the reduced light condition of videostroboscopy, which will be described later in this volume. However, the larger outside diameter increases the **risk of stimulating a gag reflex** during the study.

B. Flexible Endoscopes

Flexible endoscopes used for speech, voice, and swallowing evaluation are inserted through the **nasal cavity**. Flexible scopes differ from rigid scopes in the manner that light is transmitted through the insertion tube. Flexible scope insertion tubes contain an dense array of very small flexible **fiberoptic fibers**. These fibers are arranged so that some of them carry light to the light emitting lens and some carry light from the light pick-up lens. Each fiber presents a small dot of light to the viewing lens, the brightness and color of which is determined, in part, by the brightness and color of the light falling onto the opposite end of that

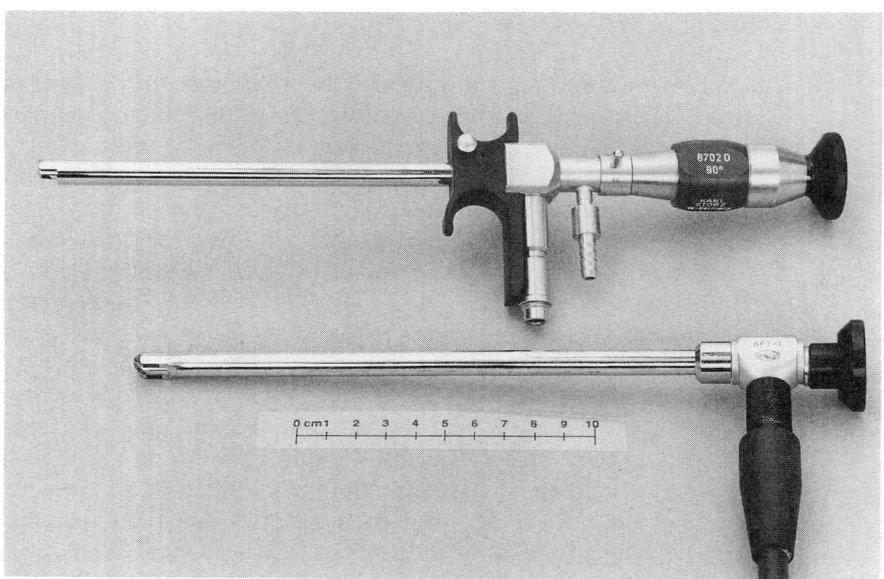

Figure 3–2. A Storz 90° (**top**) and a Nakamichi 70° (**bottom**) rigid oral endoscope.

fiber positioned at the light pick-up lens. Brightness and color are also determined by the length and quality of the fibers themselves. The result is an image that is made up of hundreds of small dots of light, similar to the halftone photographs that are published in newspapers and books.

The **advantage** of the flexible insertion tube is that **it can bend** as it is passed through the frequently irregular nasal passage, resulting in a more comfortable insertion for the patient. However, there is always some degradation of image brightness and color when reflected light is broken up and transmitted through fiberoptic fibers. Image sharpness and resolution in flexible scopes are determined by the size, quality, and density of the individual fibers within the insertion tube. Small, high quality, dense fibers provide better image resolution. However, as fiber size becomes smaller, so does the amount of light that can be transmitted through the fiber. Although fiber quality is constantly being improved, **image brightness and color representation currently are better in rigid scopes** than in flexible scopes.

Use of both end viewing and side viewing flexible endoscopes has been reported in the literature (Ibuki et al., 1982; Ibuki, Karnell, & Morris, 1983; Karnell et al., 1983). Although the relative utility of side viewing flexible endoscopes is debatable (Karnell, 1983; Shprintzen, 1983), **end viewing scopes have become the standard** due to their superior optics, image quality, and the fact that the end viewing lens provides for more controlled insertion through the nasal lumen.

II. LIGHT SOURCES

The light source is the component that provides illumination for videoendoscopy. In this section, both standard light sources, those that provide continuous light, and stroboscopic light sources will be described.

A. Standard Light Sources

Light sources provide illumination for videoendoscopy (Figure 3–3). All endoscopic light sources have several components in common. First, they contain a **lamp** which consists of a gas-filled tube and associated electrical hardware. The gases currently used

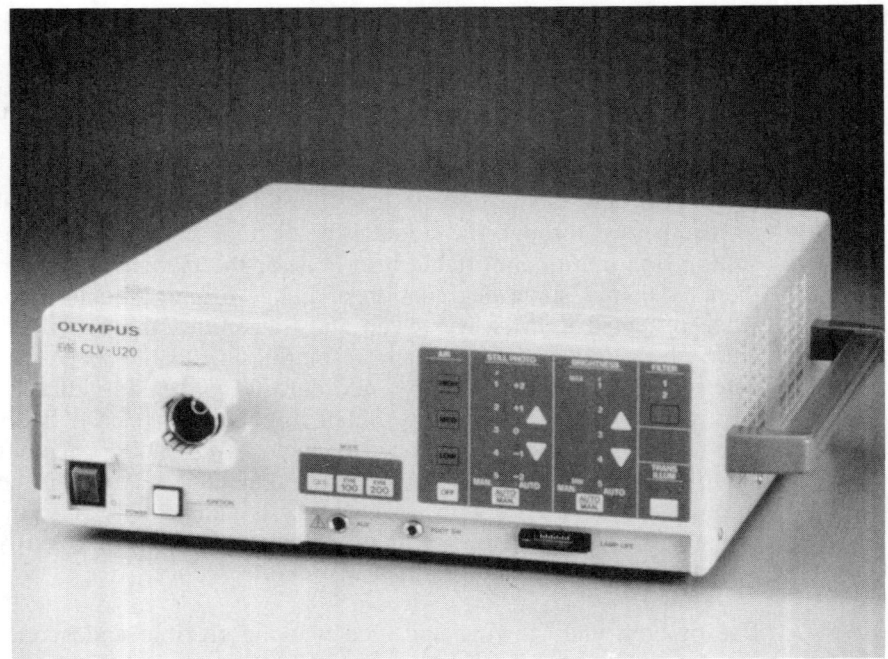

Figure 3-3. An Olympus endoscopic light source.

are predominantly **halogen** or **xenon**. When electrically charged, these gases emit a very bright light. Generally, xenon lamps provide brighter light than halogen lamps.

Another component common to all endoscopic light sources is a **fan**. The lights used in endoscopic light sources generate intense heat as well as light and therefore require cooling to prolong their life. Fans are provided to move heated air away from the light tube, thereby controlling the temperature of the tube. These fans may be very noisy or relatively quiet, depending on the type of light source used. Some stroboscopic light sources have fans that are controlled by thermostats. These fans activate when the temperature within the light source exceeds a certain limit. Most light sources use fans that run whenever the lamp is on. Light source fan noise can be important when high quality audio speech recordings during videoendoscopy are desired. It is difficult to eliminate fan noise completely from the audio recording.

B. Stroboscopic Light Sources

Special stroboscopic light sources have become popular for laryngeal videoendoscopy (Figure 3–4). These have the ability to provide standard illumination for endoscope insertion and structural evaluation and they have the added advantage of producing high intensity stroboscopic light for observation of **vocal fold vibration**. The frequency and timing of the stroboscopic effect depends on the **fundamental frequency** of the patient's voice and is controlled by the examiner, usually through a foot pedal attached to the light source.

Stroboscopic light is light that flashes on and off periodically. If we wish to observe a fast moving, quasi-periodic event like vocal fold vibration, the human visual system cannot react quickly enough for perception of vibratory activity. The edges of the vibrating vocal folds appear blurred. However, if we illuminate the vocal folds with a stroboscopic light, it is possible to create the visual perception that the rapidly moving vocal folds are moving

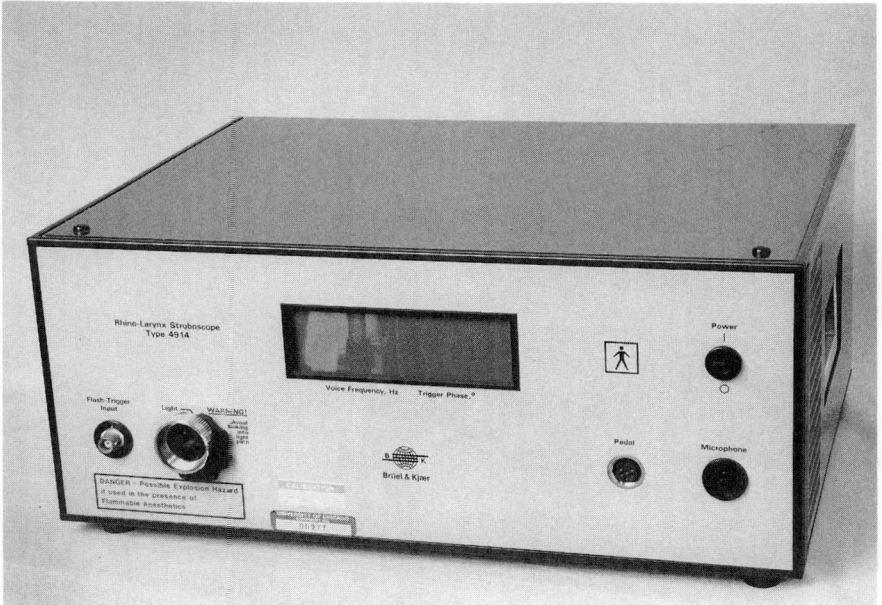

Figure 3–4. A Bruel & Kjäer stroboscopic light source. The Kay Elemetrics stroboscopic light source is shown in Figure 7–5 as part of a complete computer-supported stroboscopic recording and display system.

very slowly or not at all. For example, if we flash a light on very briefly at exactly the same time in each vocal fold vibratory cycle, what we see will appear to be motionless vocal folds. However, if we slightly change the time at which the flash occurs from one vibratory cycle to the next, we will see what appears to be slow motion (Figure 3–5).

III. CAMERAS

Improvement in videoendoscopic recording technology since the mid-1970s has been rapid and extensive. This is particularly true for video cameras. Video cameras available for videoendoscopic use were once prohibitively large, expensive, and relatively insensitive to light. With the advent of home video technology, quality has risen and costs have declined.

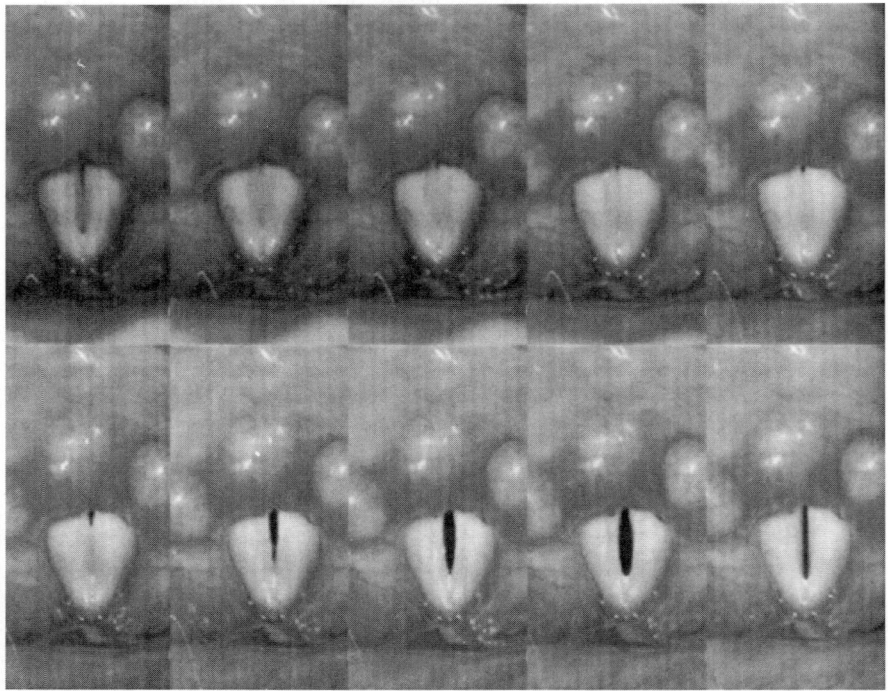

Figure 3–5. A sequence of images obtained during a stroboscopic laryngeal examination. The sequence proceeds from left to right across the top, then across the bottom of the series.

Cameras currently employed for videoendoscopy are generally of **two types**: those that contain all electronics and lenses within a **single camera unit** and those that **separate the light transducer and lens** from the power source and other electrical components of the camera (Figure 3–6). In the latter, the only part that must be handled by the examiner during the examination is the light transducer/lens component which is usually light weight (under 6 ounces) and, therefore, maneuverable when coupled with an endoscope. The self-contained units are generally less expensive and provide equally good quality recordings, but because all the electronics are included in a single unit, they are somewhat larger and heavier, requiring stabilization on the clinician's shoulder or on a tripod.

The preferred camera system is influenced by **examiner style and budget**. Some examiners prefer to work with a camera/scope arrangement that is stabilized on the examiner's shoulder or a tripod. Therefore, they prefer self-contained cameras. Others place a premium on freedom of scope maneuverability and find that dual component cameras are preferable.

IV. VIDEO RECORDERS

Analog video cassette recorders are currently the most cost-effective means of recording extended videoendoscopic images. However, now that digital audio tape recorders are available, we can expect that **digital** video tape recorders will not be far behind.

Video tape recorders used for videoendoscopy should have several features. First, a **remote control** system can be very useful for controlling the recorder during a procedure. It can be positioned within reach if the examiner is standing or sitting during the evaluation. Also, there should be a means by which recorded video tape images can be reviewed in **slow motion**. The best type of controller for slow motion review employs a round knob positioned on the front of the recorder and, depending on the model, on the remote control unit. Moreover, the slow motion should be noise free and seamless from one video field to the next. There should not be visible horizontal lines that appear as the recorder advances during slow motion. Finally, there should be a means by which **individual recorded segments can be identified** during fast-forward or fast-reverse. This is important when attempting to locate a specific segment on a given recorded video tape.

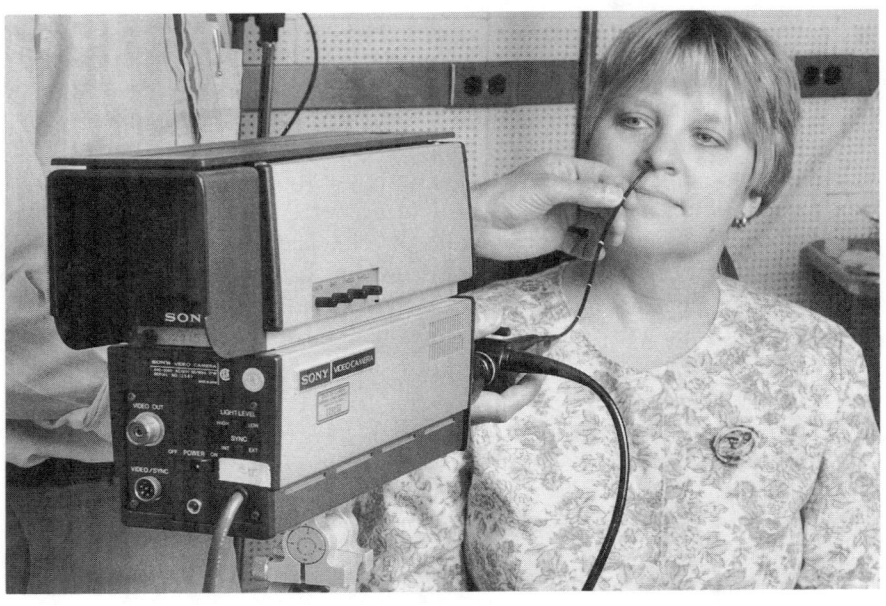

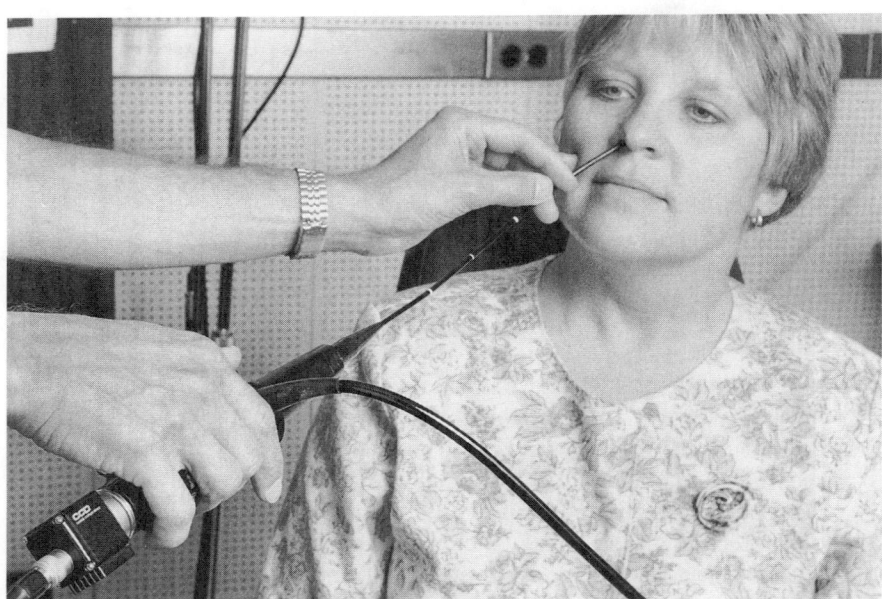

Figure 3–6. Example of a small, light-weight, hand-held electronic camera (**top**) (power source not shown) and a larger, tripod-based, tube-type camera (**bottom**).

A major consideration when designing a videoendoscopic system involves the **choice of video tape width** and therefore video cassette size that will be used. In theory, the wider the tape, the more information that can be recorded per unit space on the tape. Current choices include $\frac{3}{4}$ inch, $\frac{1}{2}$ inch, and 8 mm sizes (Figure 3–7).

A. $\frac{3}{4}$ inch

For several years, $\frac{3}{4}$ inch video cassettes were considered the best means of assuring **optimal picture quality**. The $\frac{3}{4}$ inch width made it possible to record the highest quality images possible with

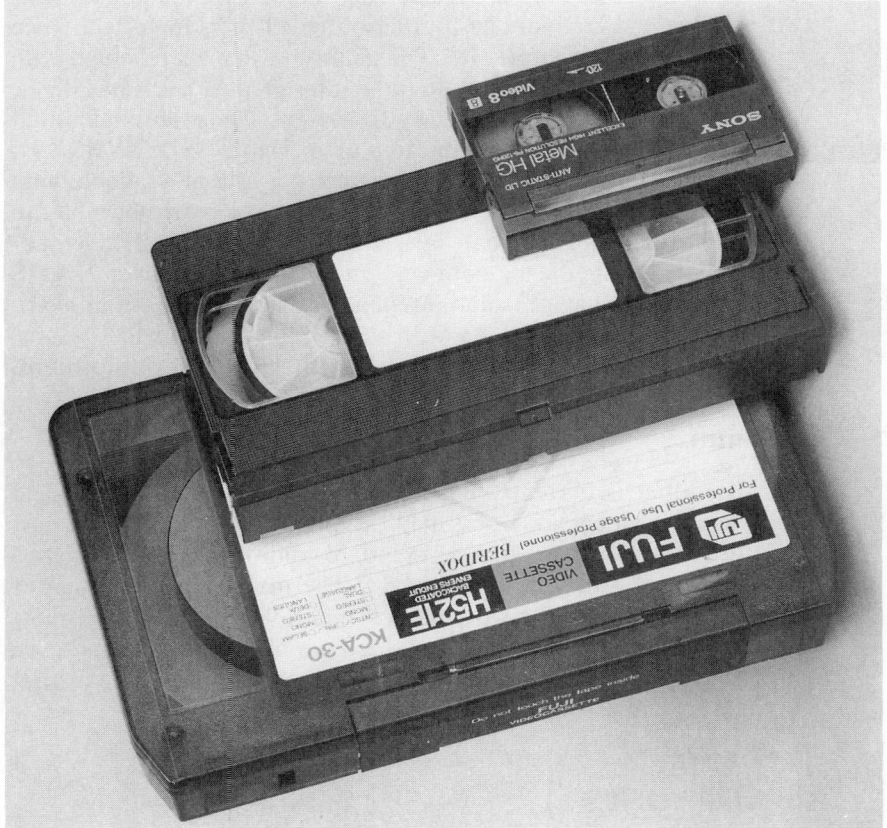

Figure 3–7. Examples of 8 mm (**top**), $\frac{1}{2}$ inch VHS (**middle**), and $\frac{3}{4}$ inch (**bottom**) videotape cassettes.

a cassette. However, these cassettes are relatively large (13.9 × 22 × 3.1 cm) and, therefore, require considerable shelf space. Cassette size can be important if all recorded studies are saved and archived because of the extensive amount of space required to store them. If storage space is limited, a smaller format cassette may be preferred.

B. $\frac{1}{2}$ inch

The $\frac{1}{2}$ inch videocassette recorders include VHS, S-VHS and Beta formats. The format most commonly used for videoendoscopy are currently **Super VHS** (S-VHS) or **standard VHS**. Both S-VHS and standard VHS cassettes are considerably smaller (10.4 × 18.7 × 2.5 cm) than $\frac{3}{4}$ inch cassettes and therefore require less storage space and are more easily transported. This is important when studies are reviewed off-site. The quality of images recorded with standard VHS recorders is slightly inferior to $\frac{3}{4}$ inch machines, but the differences are not easy to see in videoendoscopic studies and therefore may not be important. Moreover, S-VHS systems offer image resolution that is superior to that available with $\frac{3}{4}$ inch technology. However, it is important to remember that, to realize the improvement available with super VHS videorecorders, both the camera and monitor used with a S-VHS machine must have resolution equal to or better than that available from the recorder. As with most multi-component systems, **the end product is only as good as the weakest component**.

C. 8 mm

This format is currently popular in the home video market and its use for videoendoscopy may be quite acceptable. These cassettes are about the size of standard audio cassettes and thus require very little space for storage. The **major disadvantage** of this format is that the slow motion controllers available on most 8 mm machines used for home video are not as good as those on the VHS and $\frac{3}{4}$ inch machines. Use of more expensive, industrial grade machines may overcome this limitation.

V. MICROPHONES

Two types of microphones are employed during videoendoscopy. Traditional microphones are used to transduce the patient's and clinician's voices for the videotape record. Contact microphones are used during videostroboscopy to synchronize the flash rate of the stroboscopic light source with the rate of the patient's vocal fold vibration.

A. Traditional Microphones

Among the most important benefits of videoendoscopic evaluation of speech is that it enables simultaneous sound and visual recording. Given that speech is an acoustic phenomenon, the quality of the sound recording must be high. For this reason, careful consideration is necessary when selecting a microphone. A wide variety of high quality microphones is commercially available. In general, the microphone chosen for videoendoscopic examinations should be of similar quality to those used for high quality audio recordings of speech.

Microphone position during the study can be very important. A boom-mounted microphone system is usually adequate because videoendoscopic procedures impose certain restrictions on patient head mobility. However, it is important that the mouth-to-microphone distance be adjusted so that the acoustic speech signal can be picked up adequately. Because light sources usually have cooling fans that produce a certain amount of noise, it is important that the microphone placement avoids such background noise that interferes with speech recording. We have found that a **headmounted microphone is optimal** (Figure 3–8). Such microphones allow constant, close positioning of the microphone to the patient's mouth regardless how the patient's head may move during the procedure.

B. Contact Microphones

The contact microphone used for videostroboscopy is placed over the **thyroid lamina lateral to the midline** of the patient's **anterior neck**. It may be held in place manually by the patient, but usually it is secured with a neck strap (Figure 3–9).

Contact microphones used with most stroboscopic light sources consist of a stethoscope-like diaphragm housing connected to the light source with an air-filled tube. The contact microphone diaphragm must be held against the neck tissue with sufficient force to permit tissue vibrations of the neck associated with voice to be picked up by the diaphragm which converts the mechanical

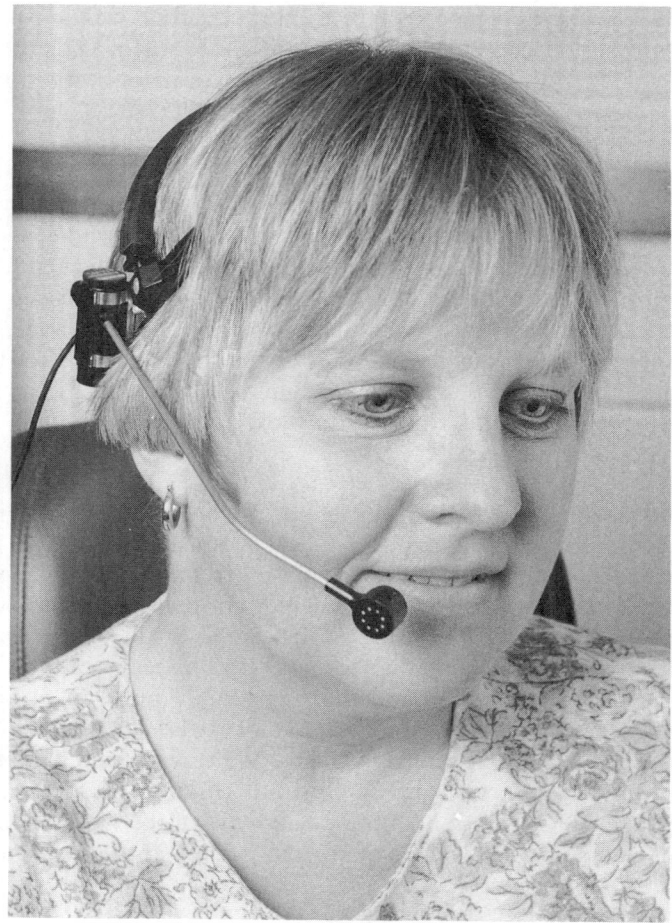

Figure 3–8. A head-mounted microphone.

tissue vibrations back into acoustic energy like the skin of a drum. If the microphone is not held firmly against the neck, the diaphragm will not complete the transduction process adequately and the stroboscopic light source will not flash at the desired rate, and, depending on the type of light source, may not flash at all. The clinician must carefully position the contact microphone so that it is functioning properly prior to endoscope insertion.

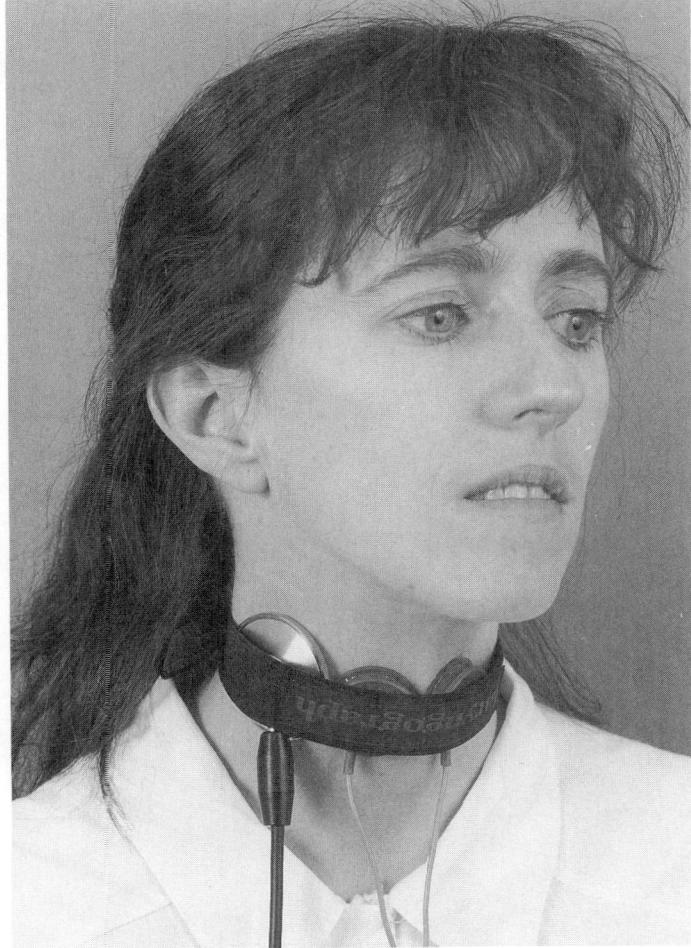

Figure 3–9. A stroboscopic contact microphone held in place with a neck strap that is also used to position electroglottographic electrodes.

The acoustic energy from the diaphragm is transmitted via the air-filled tube to a microphone housed within the stroboscopic light source. It is here that the acoustic energy is transduced into electrical impulses used to control the rate of stroboscopic light flashing.

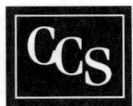

CHAPTER

4

Velopharyngeal Videoendoscopy

The details of scope insertion and manipulation will be described in this chapter. Special considerations regarding patient preparation, management, and positioning will be discussed.

It should be clear that several approaches to videoendoscopic examination are possible, and the choice of approach depends on the purpose of the procedure. Generally, videoendoscopic procedures for assessment of speech physiology attempt to provide physiologic information about either **velopharyngeal or laryngeal function** during speech production.

Whether the purpose is to evaluate the velopharynx or larynx, or whether the approach is oral or nasal, a thorough understanding of the **surface anatomy and physiology** is necessary. Those interested in performing the procedure must have expertise regarding the area to be examined. How such expertise is acquired varies and may involve a mix of didactic and practical experiences. Currently, there is no recognized course of study designed to qualify an individual to perform endoscopy, although there is consensus that some level of graduate training is necessary. The nature and duration of training is subject to considerable debate.

Knowledge of and adherence to "**Universal Precautions**" for handling and sterilized equipment used for endoscopy is critical. A review of these precautions is provided in Appendix A. Since implementation of these precautions varies among institutions, it is necessary that the quidelines determined by the institution where the procedure is to be performed be understood and followed. **There can be absolutely no compromise where patient safety is concerned.**

I. VELOPHARYNGEAL PROCEDURES

Both nasal and oral endoscopic procedures can be useful for evaluation of velopharyngeal physiology. Therefore, detailed procedures for performing both will be considered here.

A. Velopharyngeal Videoendoscopy—Nasal Approach

Videoendoscopic assessment of velopharyngeal physiology is most frequently performed with a flexible fiberoptic endoscope inserted through the nasal passages. The **task requires special knowledge and skills**. Nasal anatomy and physiology are somewhat variable among patients. There is no substitute for clear understanding of both normal and abnormal nasal anatomy and physiology. The nasal passages are lined with mucosa containing both surface and deep sensory receptors and, therefore, may be quite sensitive to **tactile stimulation**. Moreover, the nasal lining is highly vascular. Traumatic impact between an endoscope and the nasal mucosa can result in **bleeding**. Finally, the risks of **disease transmission** must be well understood and minimized or eliminated.

1. Patient Preparation

Preparing a patient for nasal endoscopy is an exercise in **minimizing patient discomfort** and **maximizing cooperation**. In the majority of adult cases, patient discomfort is negligible, and cooperation is excellent. Usually, the adult patient is concerned about her or his voice or resonance problem and, therefore, motivated to cooperate. Also, since the nasal lumen in adults can usually accomodate a 3.6 mm diameter flexible endoscopic insertion tube, potential for nasal discomfort is relatively small. However, there are adults who bring considerable **anxiety** to the videoendoscopic procedure and some have unusually **small nasal passages**. In children, anxiety and small nasal passages are the norm. These issues can be managed through the cautious use of smaller endoscopes, topical anesthesia, vasoconstrictive, agents, and psycho-behavioral manipulation.

a. Anesthesia and Vasoconstriction

Topical anesthetics reduce surface tactile sensation in nasal mucous membrane. Some mild topical anesthetics sold without prescription are used orally for tooth pain. Those used for endoscopy are not available over the counter.

Vasoconstrictors temporarily restrict blood supply to the affected area, resulting in temporary shrinking of nasal mucosa. Commonly known nonprescription vasoconstrictors include **Afrin®** and **Neosynephrine®**.

The use of anesthesia in preparation for nasal endoscopy is very common, although not universal. Given what is known about the sensitivity of the lining of the nasal passages to tactile stimulation, it seems intuitive that some measure of nasal anesthesia should be not only preferred but demanded by the patient. This, however, is not the case. The application of **nasal anesthesia can itself be a noxious stimulus**. For some patients, application of the anesthesia and the resulting sensations are more objectionable than the insertion of the endoscope without anesthesia. It is quite reasonable to let the **patient's preference** guide the use of anesthesia. However, it is the clinician's responsibility to stop the procedure and apply anesthesia if the patient becomes uncomfortable during an unanesthetized procedure. It does no good to complete a procedure when there is a risk that patient discomfort may jeopardize the validity of the findings.

Common anesthetic agents used topically for nasal endoscopy include **4% lidocaine** (.04 gm/100 ml solution), **2% pontocaine** (.02 gm/100 ml solution), and **4% cocaine** (.04 gm/100 ml solution). All three are very effective. Cocaine has the added benefit of being a vasoconstrictor as well as anesthetic. It has the much more important limitation of being a substance that is frequently abused. For this reason, it is advisable to avoid use of cocaine for routine nasal endoscopic speech evaluations.

In general, only the **smallest amount of anesthesia necessary** to produce the desired effect should be used for nasal endoscopy. The minimal amount of anesthesia for adequate effect varies with the size of the patient. No more than **three sprays** from a standard manual atomizer are usually necessary to provide the desired effect in any patient.

When applying anesthesia with a standard manual atomizer, **an average of 0.12 ml solution is provided for each complete spray**. Three sprays would provide an average of 14 mg anesthesia. In children, the maximum single dose of viscous lidocaine should not exceed 5 mg/kg body weight (Smith, R. M., 1980). In the case of 4% lidocaine, this amounts to 70 mg for a child weighing 14 kg (30 lbs). Assuming that everything sprayed is absorbed by the patient, 14 mg represents 20% or one fifth of the maximum recommended dose for a child this size. For an average adult weighing 70 kg, this would amount to 3% or one thirty-third of the maximum recommended dose. It is virtually impossible, therefore, to exceed the maximum recommended dose of 4% lidocaine if no more than three sprays from a hand held atomizer are provided (Figure 4–1).

The **risk of allergic reaction** to topical anesthetics applied in the quantities needed for nasal videoendoscopy is small but real. It is advisable, therefore, to provide nasal anesthesia only with the approval of qualified medical personnel in a facility that is prepared to respond to the most unusual patient reaction.

Use of vasoconstriction is also optional in many patients. However, in patients with hypertrophic turbinates or a deviated septum, **vasoconstriction may be essential** and therefore should be available. In some patients vasoconstrictors have a profound effect on nasal mucosa and significantly increase the nasal lumen (Figure 4–2).

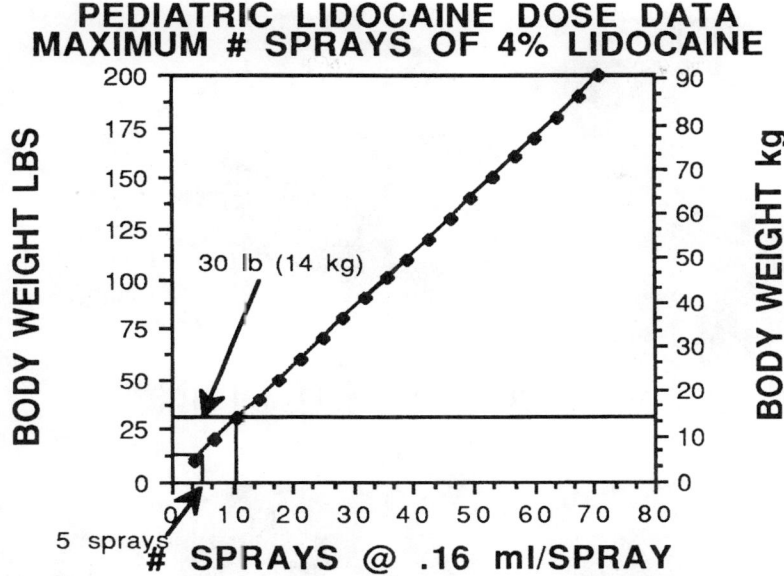

PEDIATRIC LIDOCAINE DOSE DATA
MAXIMUM # SPRAYS OF 4% LIDOCAINE

Figure 4–1. Maximum dosage of 4% lidocaine (at 0.16 ml/spray from a hand-held atomizer) for children by body weight. Note that 5 sprays represent only 50% of the maximum dose for a 30 pound (14 kg) child.

Application of nasal anesthetics and vasoconstriction with an atomizer can be particularly **noxious to children** (Figure 4–3). In such cases, special procedures for applying the material may be in order. One approach is to use **cotton pledgets** (strips of cotton material) that are saturated with a controlled amount of solution. These pledgets can be gradually introduced into the nasal passage until completely packed without causing discomfort to the patient. Bayonet forceps are useful for moving the pledget into the anterior nares. Care must be taken to avoid contacting the patient directly with the forceps, and under no circumstances should the forceps be inserted into the nasal cavity beyond the nares. Skillful application of **behavioral management techniques** similar to those used in speech therapy is very useful.

b. Behavioral Management
Behavioral management techniques are sometimes useful when the patient is anxious about nasal videoendoscopy.

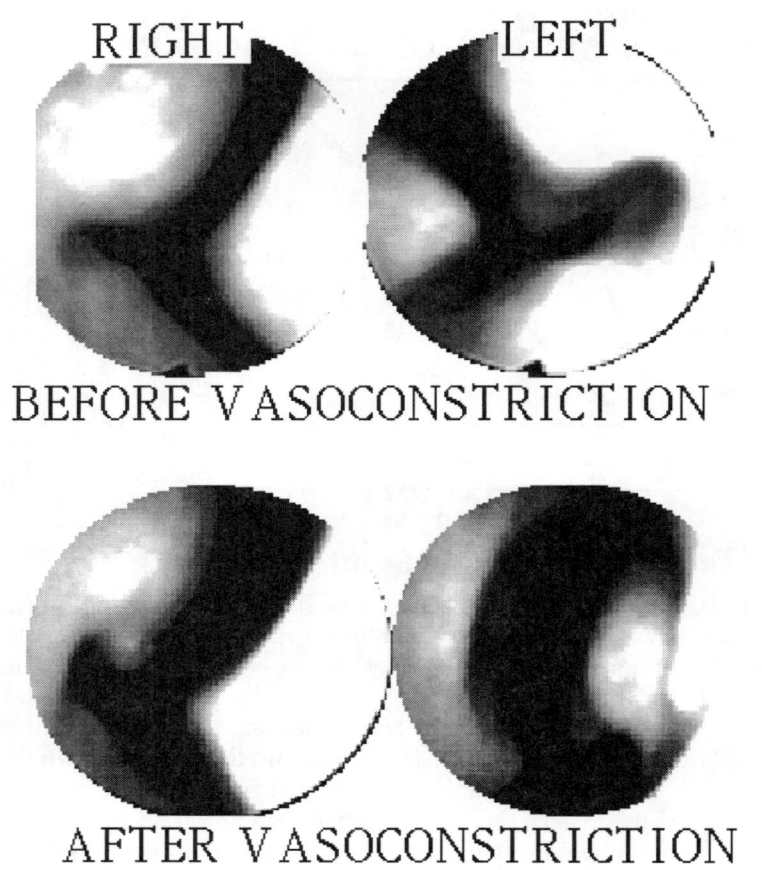

RIGHT   LEFT

BEFORE VASOCONSTRICTION

AFTER VASOCONSTRICTION

Figure 4–2. Application of vasoconstrictor may increase the nasal lumen.

Frequently, verbal assurance is adequate to win the confidence and cooperation of the anxious patient. In adults, it is frequently useful to explain that, because the procedure is a speech evaluation, it is important that the patient be as comfortable as possible throughout the study. An uncomfortable patient will have difficulty producing normal, natural speech during the procedure. Therefore, while a medical examination must place patient comfort second to the diagnosis of disease, the speech evaluation must make **patient comfort the top priority**. Moreover,

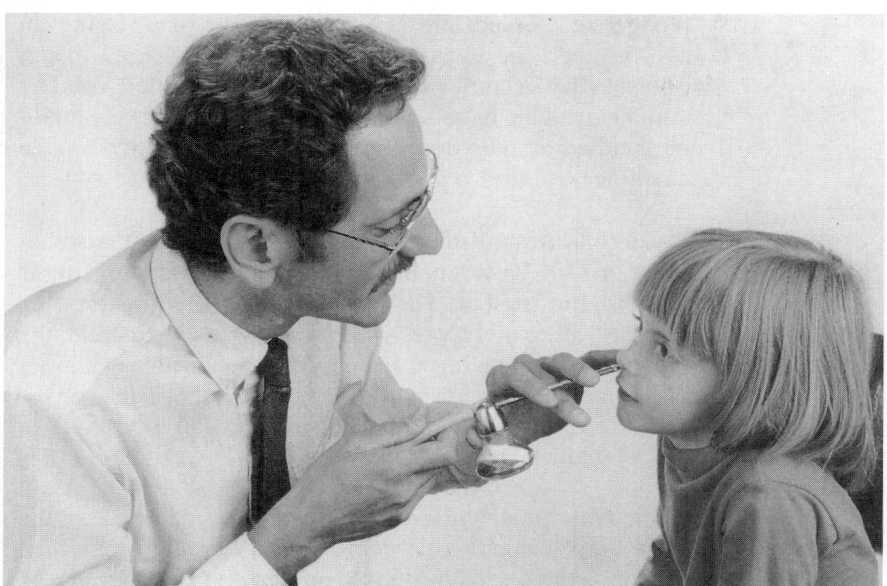

Figure 4–3. A hand-held atomizer is useful for applying small doses of topical anesthesia or vasoconstrictor.

it is important to assure the adult patient that it is important to the success of the examination for the examiner to be told if there is discomfort during the evaluation.

Managing children can require a much more organized approach. It is advantageous if the child has not had experience with endoscopic procedures and has no preconceived notions about what will happen. In such patients, it is frequently beneficial to **appeal to the child's interest in the television equipment**. Children enjoy pushing the buttons that turn on the machines and seeing themselves on the video monitor. It is a good idea to start by recording a head-and-shoulders view of the child while he or she is saying their name, repeating some simple sentences (preferably those that will be used during the evaluation), and answering some simple questions. It is useful to elicit a conversational speech sample if possible.

Small **children enjoy helping with the nasal pledget preparation**. The examiner may demonstrate how a pledget is cut and allow the child to cut one. Using an eye dropper, the examiner may demonstrate how to apply anesthesia and vasoconstrictor to the pledget. The child may then have a turn at this. This process should be handled as play and represents an opportunity for the examiner to build rapport with the child (Figure 4–4).

During insertion of the pledget into the nostril, it is sometimes **useful to have the child place an index finger next to the nostril**. The examiner may then instruct the child to alternately press the nostril closed to hold the pledget, and then release the nostril when the examiner is prepared to advance the pledget further. This serves, again, to keep the child cooperating and involved in the procedure.

Also, with small children, the examiner may ask if the child knows what a periscope is. The examiner may then introduce the **endoscope as a special type of periscope** where you look through one side to see what is at the other. The child then may be permitted to look through the endoscope. After the scope is attached to the video camera, the examiner can show the child how anything that is placed near the lighted tip of the scope appears on the video monitor. The examiner may demonstrates how this works with a button or design on the child's shirt, then the child's finger, then the mouth, and perhaps the nose.

Most children are interested and frequently amused to see the **movement of the flexible tip** of the flexible endoscope insertion tube. The child may be encouraged to gently touch the insertion tube and may be permitted to move the control bar that bends the insertion tube tip.

It may be useful to explain to the child prior to insertion that the purpose of the study is to **"find the trap door"** (velopharyngeal port) in the back of the child's nose. Most children know what a "trap door" is or can easily understand when an explanation is offered. The child is then asked to help watch for the trap door on the video monitor.

Just prior to attempting insertion, it is advisable to place the insertion tube, approximately 1 cm from the tip so as

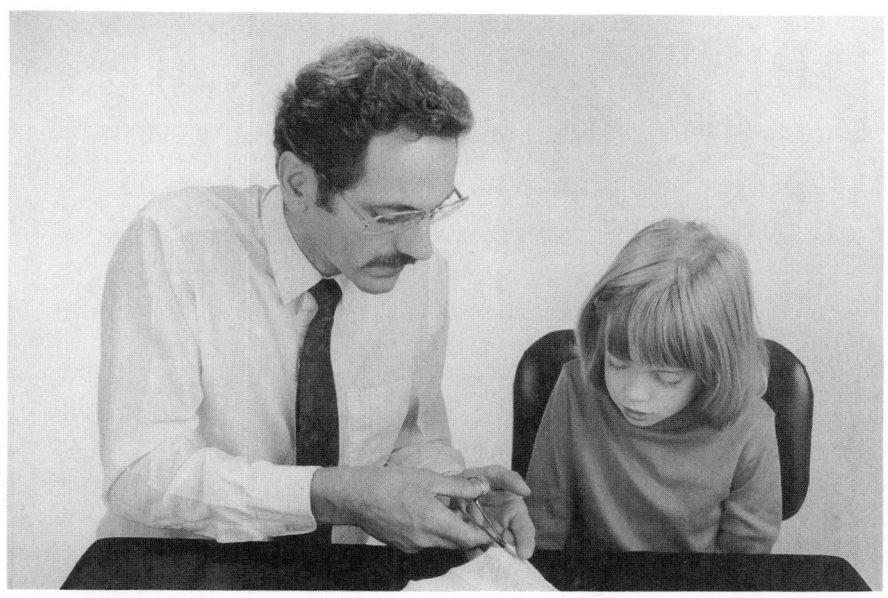

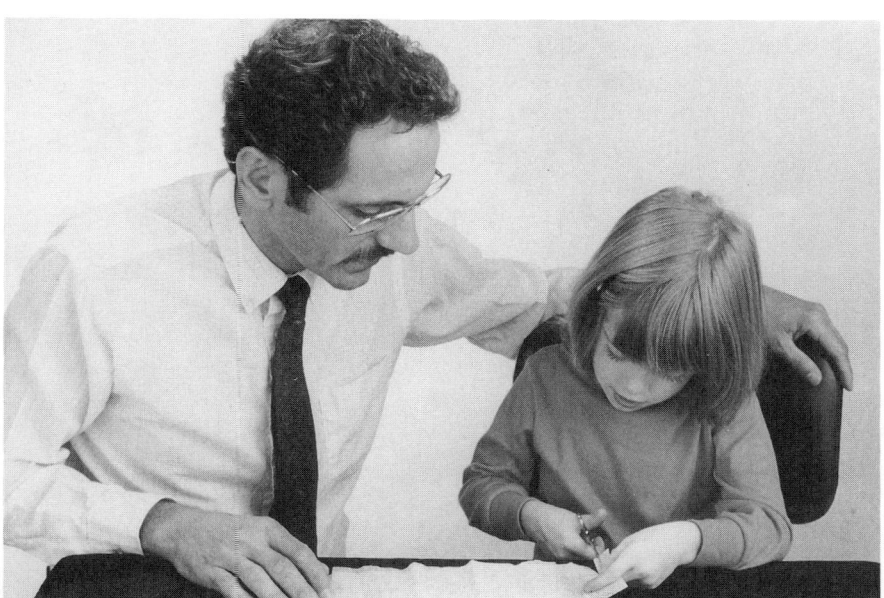

Figure 4–4. Preparation and careful application of a nasal pledget soaked with anesthesia and vasoconstrictor may be more acceptable by small children and provides an opportunity to build rapport. *(continued)*

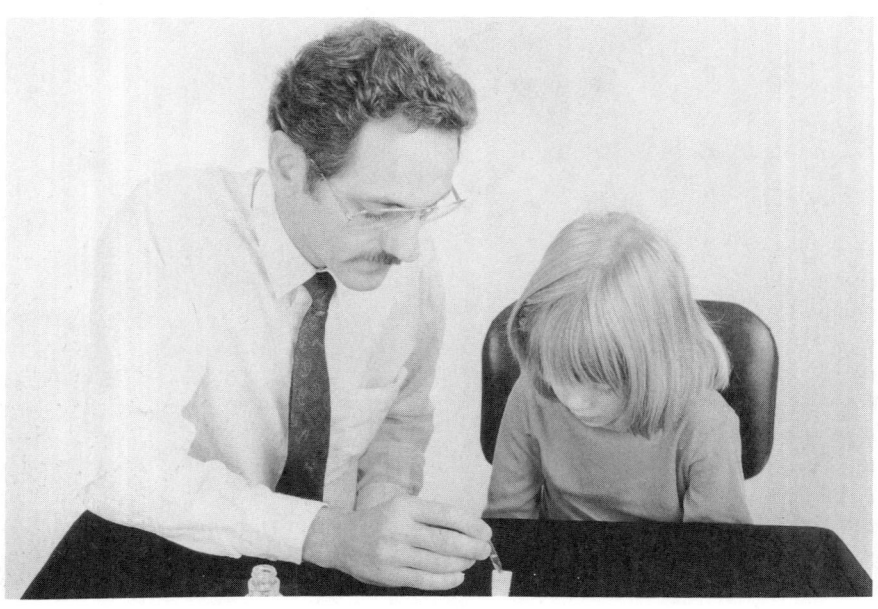

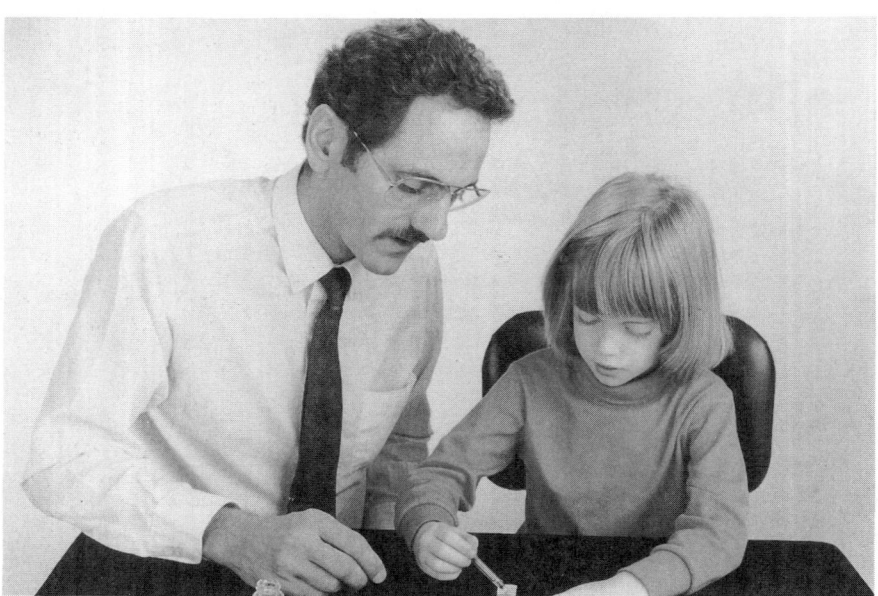

Figure 4–4 *(continued)*

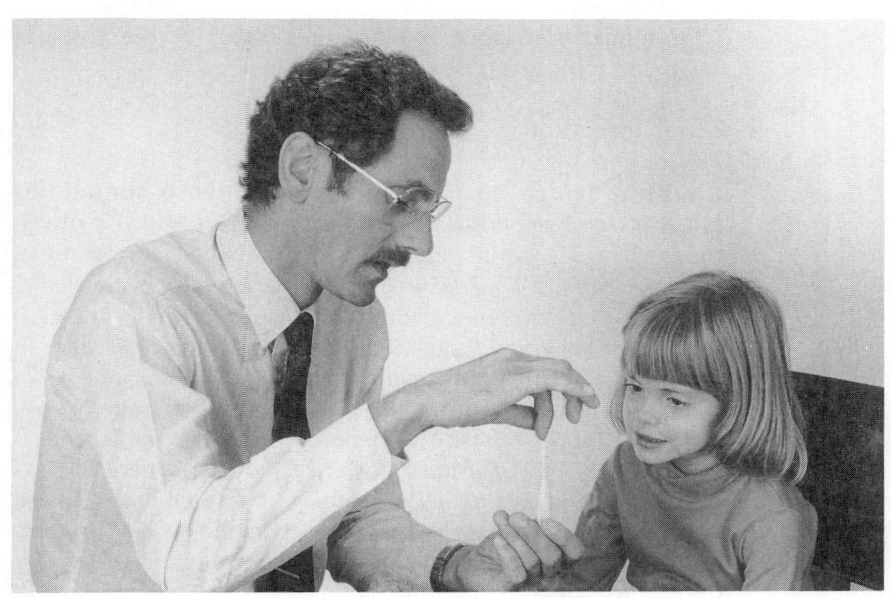

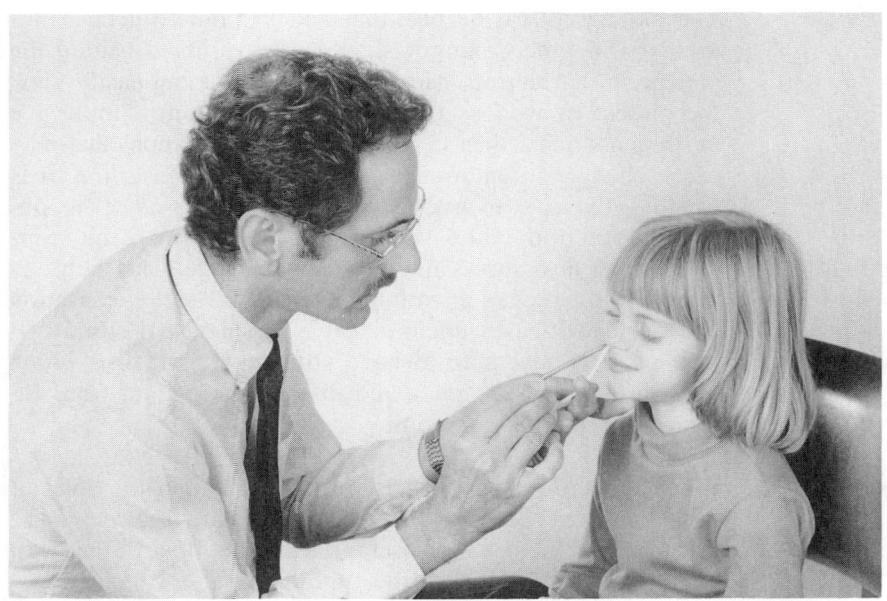

Figure 4–4 *(continued)*

not to foul the lens, in **surgical lubricant**. This will help minimize resistance between the scope and the surfaces of the nasal cavity during insertion.

2. Nasal Insertion

Choosing which nostril to attempt insertion is **sometimes arbitrary** and sometimes determined by the **patient's physiology**. In cases of unlateral cleft lip and palate, for example, the nasal septum is always deviated toward the noncleft side. This usually results in a significantly larger lumen on the cleft side. Insertion should, therefore, begin with the cleft side. In noncleft or bilateral cleft patients, the choice may not be so clear. Visual inspection of the anterior nasal passages is not always helpful because the lumen may appear large anteriorly but may be constricted posteriorly. If the patient has experienced nasal endoscopy previously, it may be useful to ask which side was evaluated and whether there was any discomfort. Patients usually remember if there was any difficulty during insertion.

The patient should be positioned facing the clinician (Figure 4–5). A video monitor should be positioned behind the patient so that during insertion the clinician can easily view the patient as well as the video monitor using simple eye movements rather than head or upper body rotations that may cause changes in endoscope position. During insertion, it is usually advisable to ask the patient, child or adult, to **observe a second video screen** positioned behind the clinician which also shows the endoscopic image. This helps to remove the patient's attention from internal tactile sensation and, instead focuses attention on external visual stimuli. It may also be advisable to have **soft music playing** which may further serve to relax and distract the patient from focusing on internal sensation.

When the tip of the scope is positioned within the anterior nasal chamber just behind the nostril, it is advisable to pause and visualize the inferior nasal turbinate; the floor of the nasal cavity; and, if possible, the middle nasal turbinate. This **serves to orient the examiner** and provides an opportunity to quickly **evaluate the size of the anterior lumen of the nasal passage**. If the turbinates appear enlarged and the

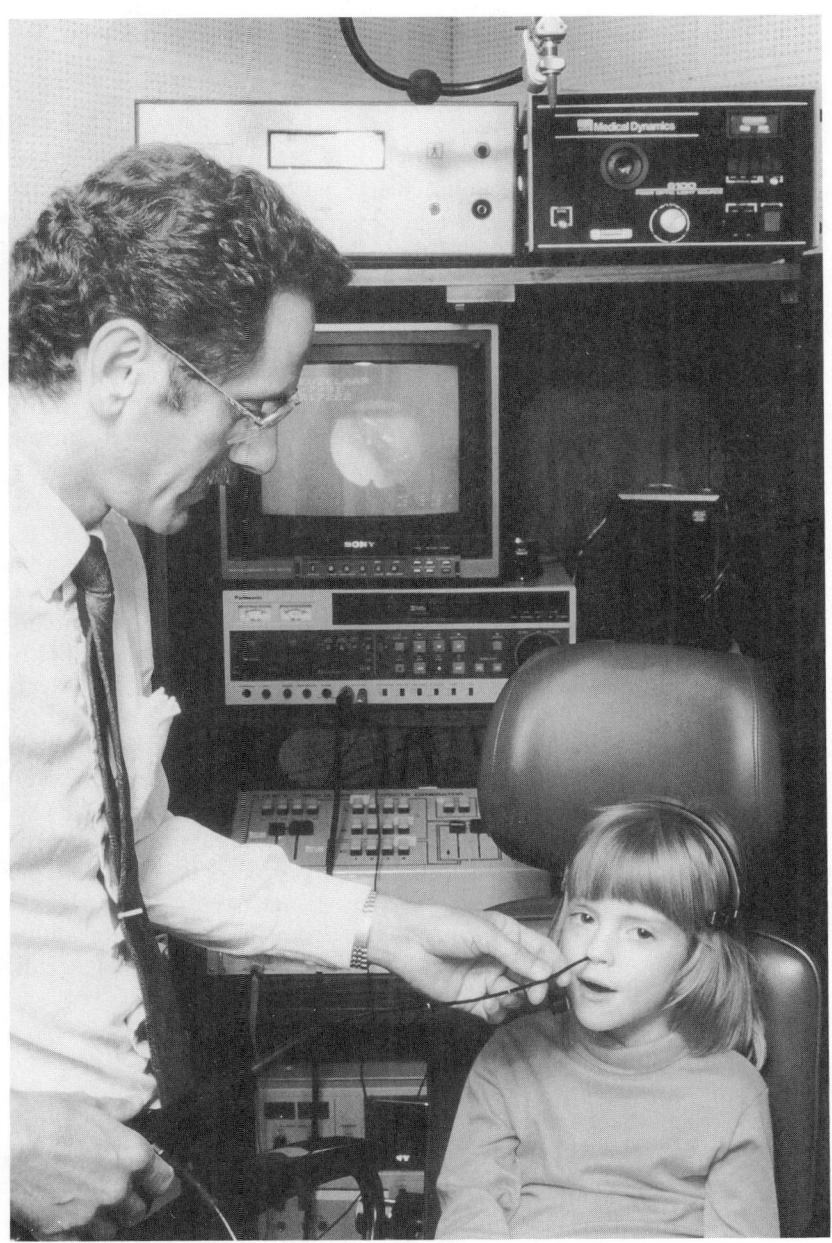

Figure 4–5. A patient positioned for nasal videoendoscopy.

lumen small, the examiner should elect to withdraw the scope and either apply additional vasoconstriction or defer to the opposite side.

If the middle turbinate can be visualized, the examiner may advance the scope sloping slightly upward toward the middle turbinate, taking care to pause before making contact. By adjusting the insertion tube tip control arm to cause a slight downward bend in the tip of the scope, the middle nasal meatus should come into view. The middle meatus is the space between the nasal septum, the inferior nasal turbinate, and the middle nasal turbinate. If the middle meatus appears large enough to accommodate the scope, the examiner may gently advance the insertion tube (Figure 4–6). It is frequently useful to have the patient begin to **produce a speech sample** at this time which may further distract the patient from focusing on internal nasal sensation.

Movement through the middle meatus should be a smooth, gentle, horizontal gesture. The examiner should be sensitive to the slightest resistance to movement through the lumen. **If resistance is encountered**, the examiner must quickly decide whether to **proceed, pause**, or **withdraw**. This decision is based on whether and how the patient may have reacted to the stimulus. It is not uncommon that some resistance perceived by the examiner does not result in any sensation for the patient, particularly if topical anesthetics are in use. However, given sufficient pressure, the patient will report sensation. The examiner must be prepared to withdraw the scope in favor of an altered approach at any time there is risk of generating a strong response from the patient. In adults, middle nasal meatus insertion is nearly always successful. Success in children is less frequent.

If insertion through the middle nasal meatus is not possible or seems likely to generate discomfort for the patient, the examiner may choose to **withdraw the scope to the anterior nasal chamber**, redirect the tip of the scope downward until the floor of the nasal passage becomes visible and the inferior nasal meatus becomes visible. Advancing through the inferior meatus (Figure 4–7) should proceed similarly to advancing through the middle nasal meatus. If insertion through either middle or inferior passages is not possible, the

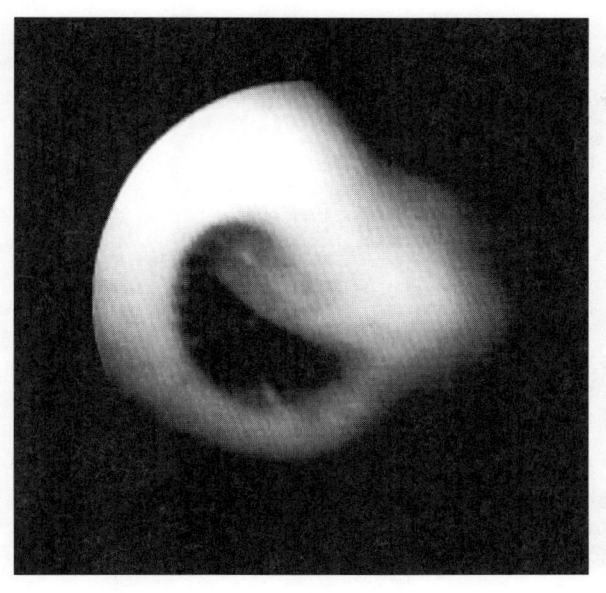

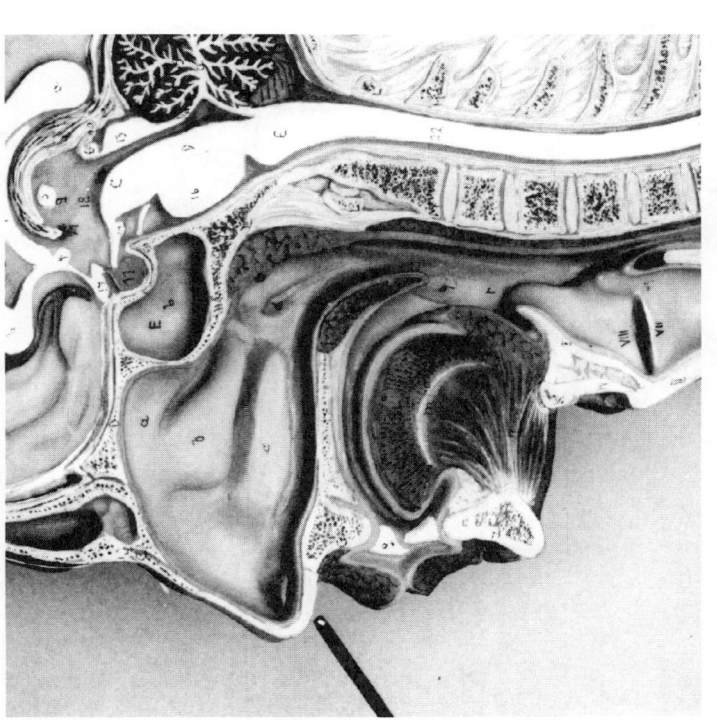

Figure 4–6. A flexible endoscope is shown at various points during insertion through the middle nasal meatus. Endoscopic images show typical views through the endoscope at each position. *(continued)*

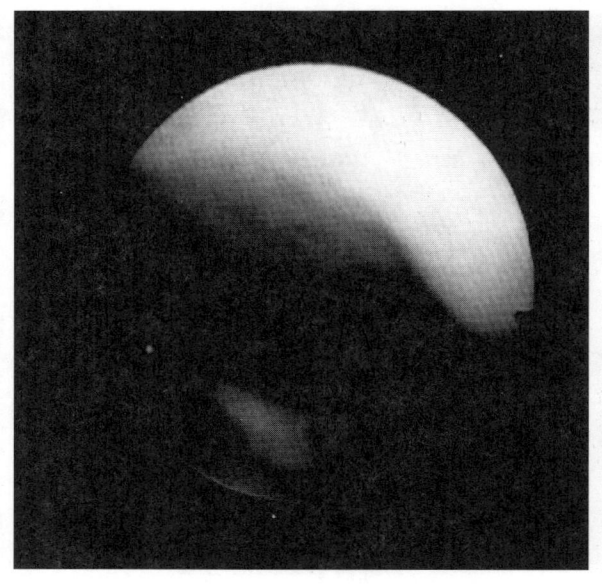

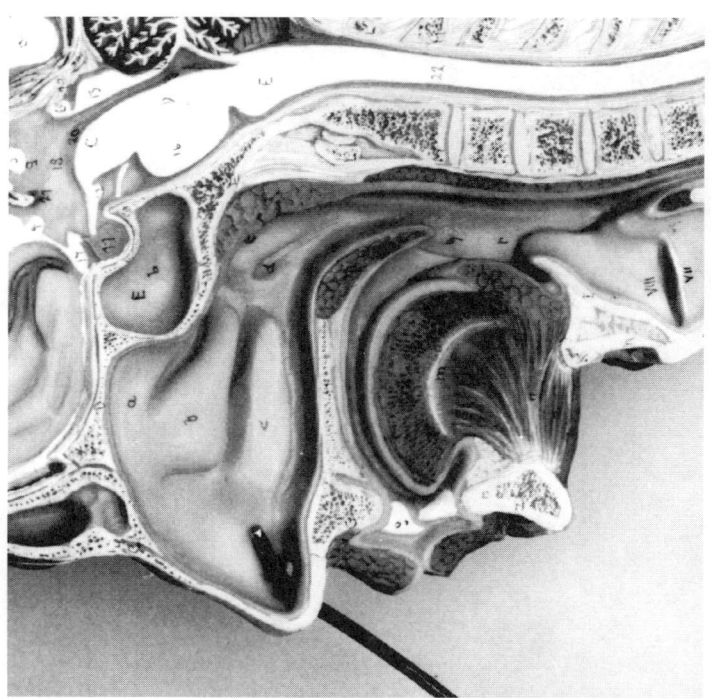

Figure 4–6. Views from a flexible endoscope *(continued)*

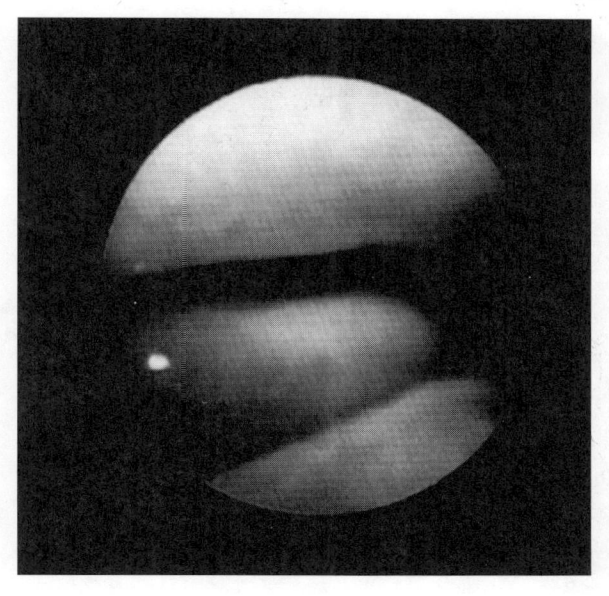

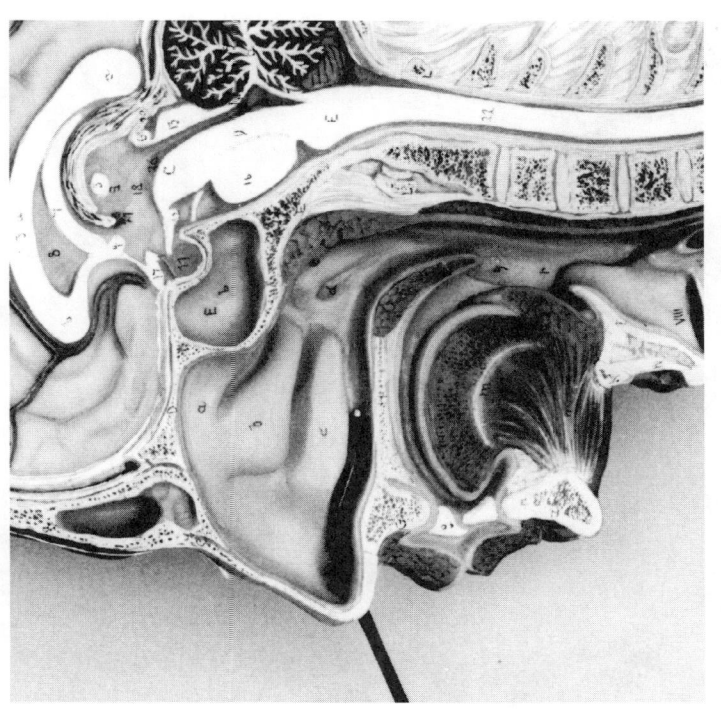

Figure 4–6. Views from a flexible endoscope *(continued)*

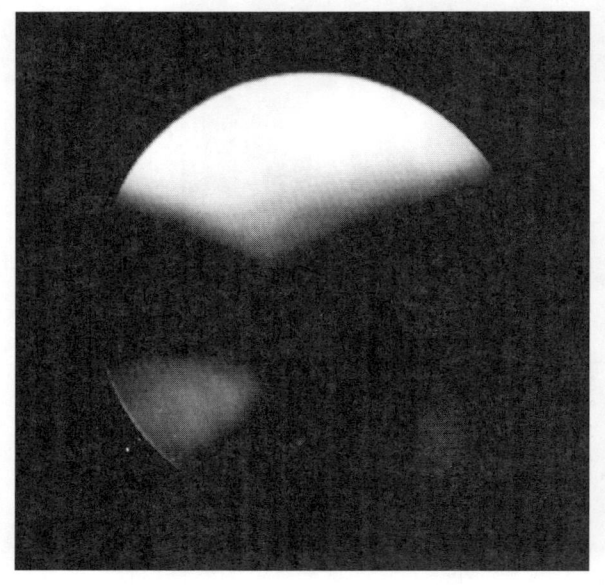

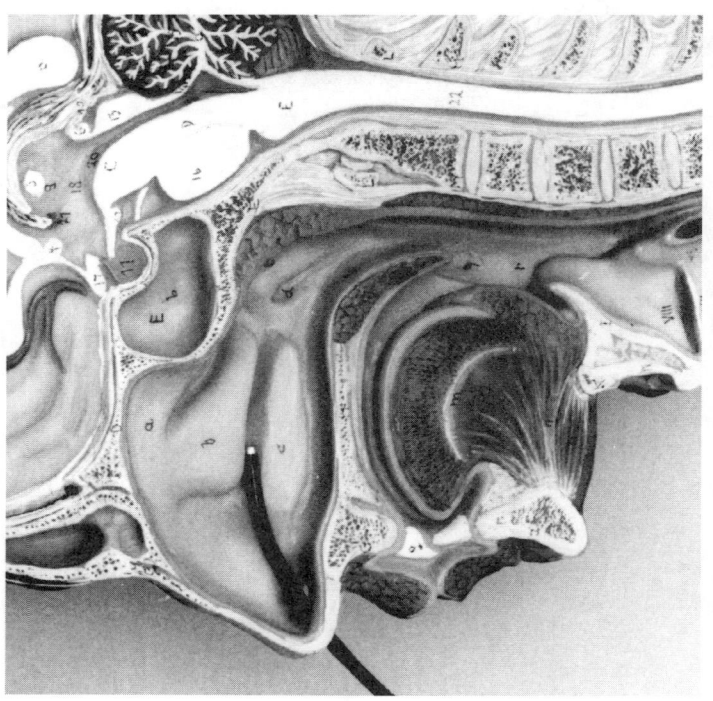

Figure 4–6. Views from a flexible endoscope *(continued)*

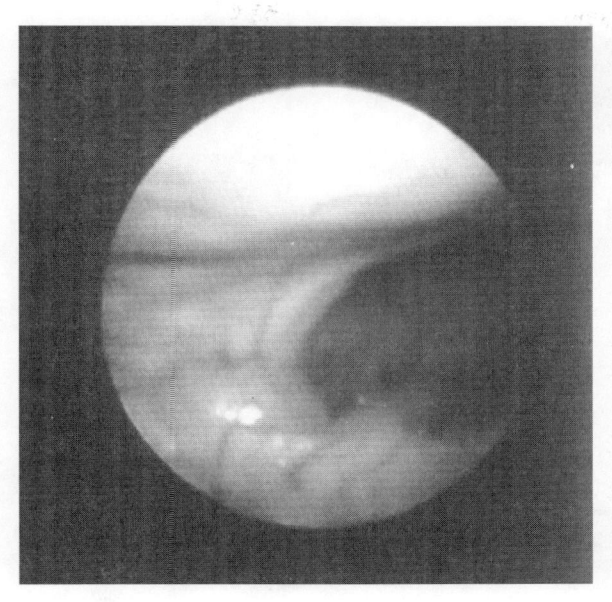

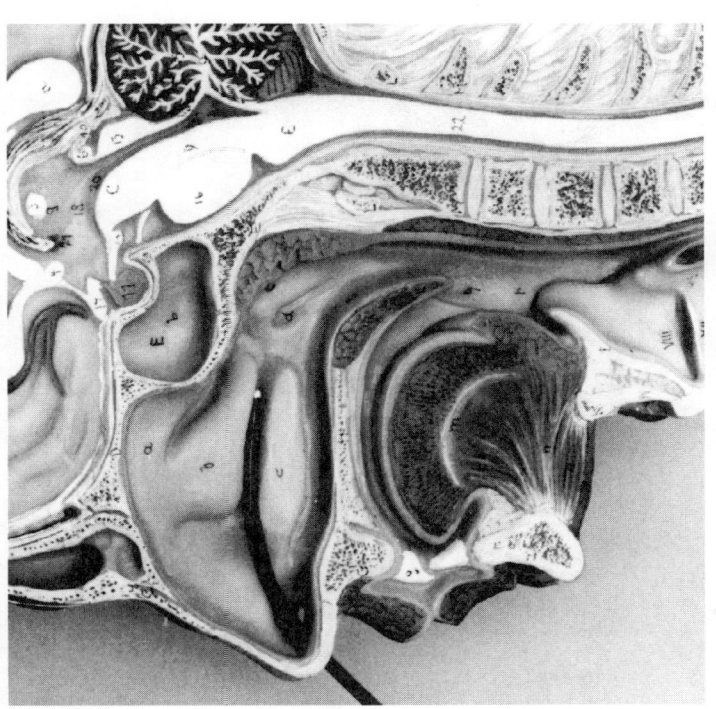

Figure 4–6. Views from a flexible endoscope *(continued)*

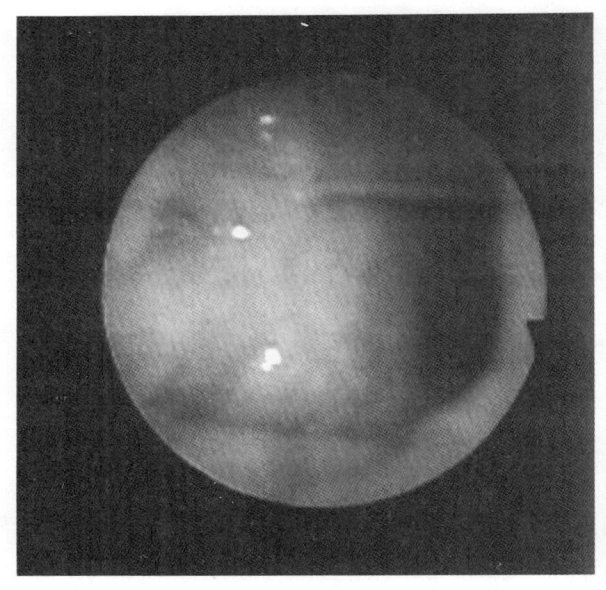

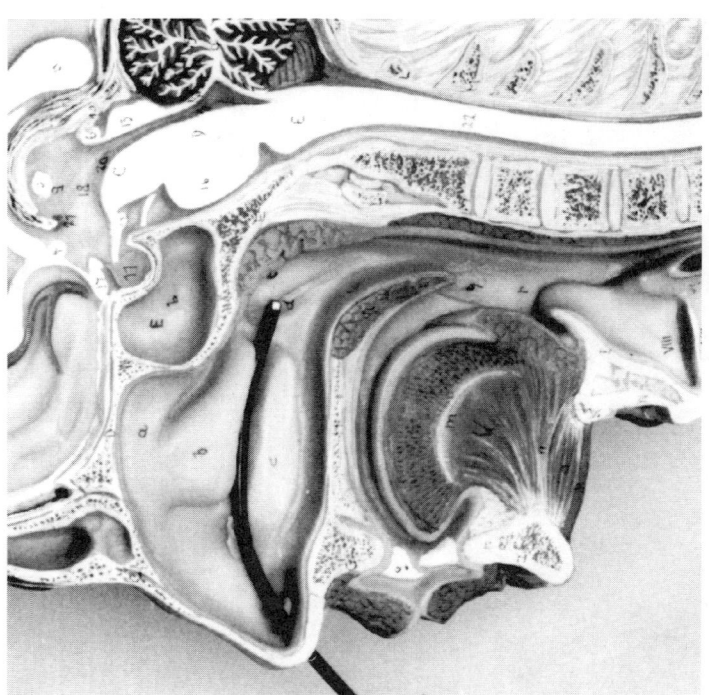

Figure 4–6. Views from a flexible endoscope *(continued)*

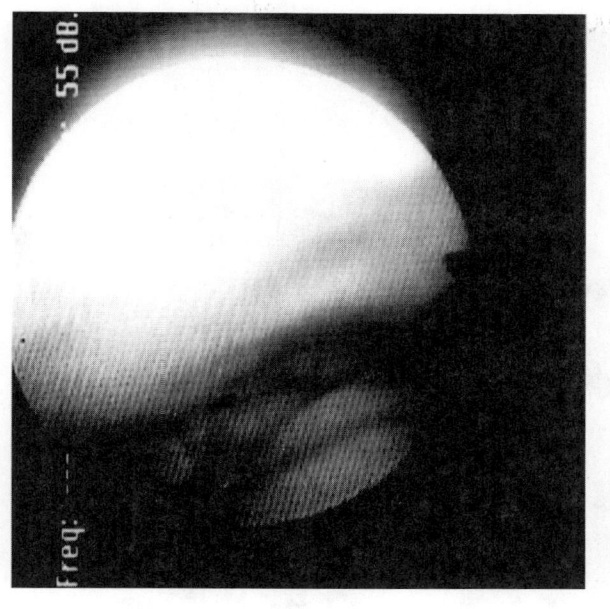

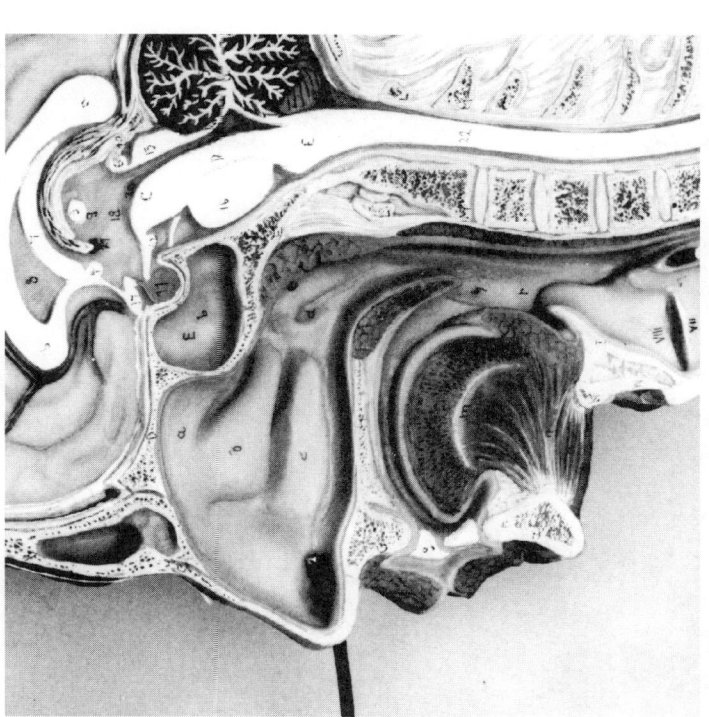

Figure 4–7. A flexible endoscope is shown at various points during insertion through the inferior nasal meatus. Endoscopic images show typical views through the endoscope at each position.

63

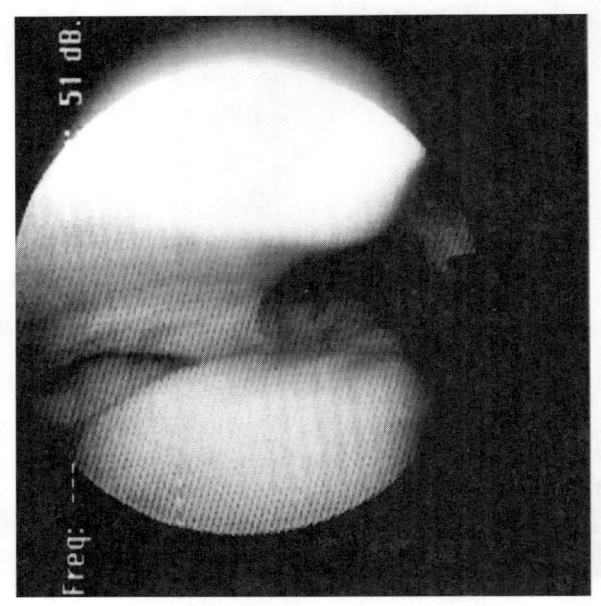

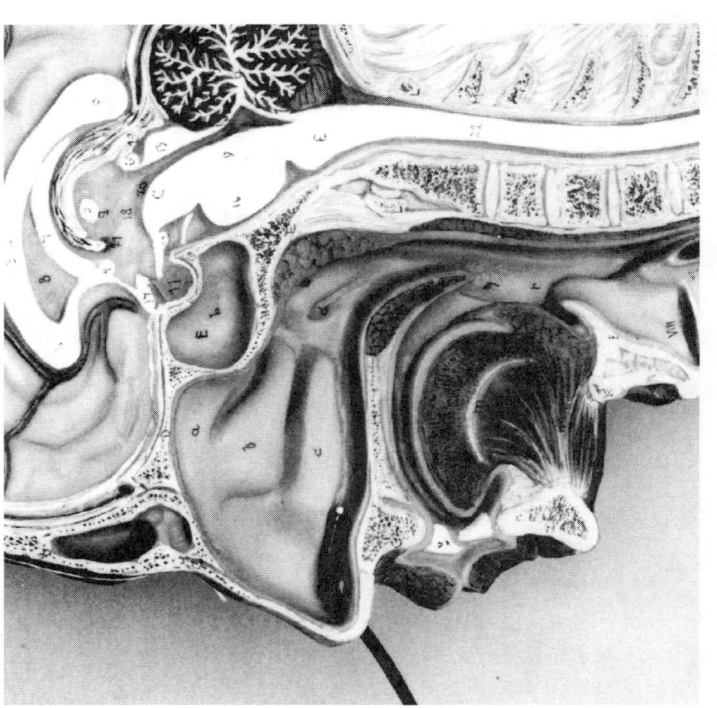

Figure 4–7. Views from insertion through the inferior nasal meatus *(continued)*

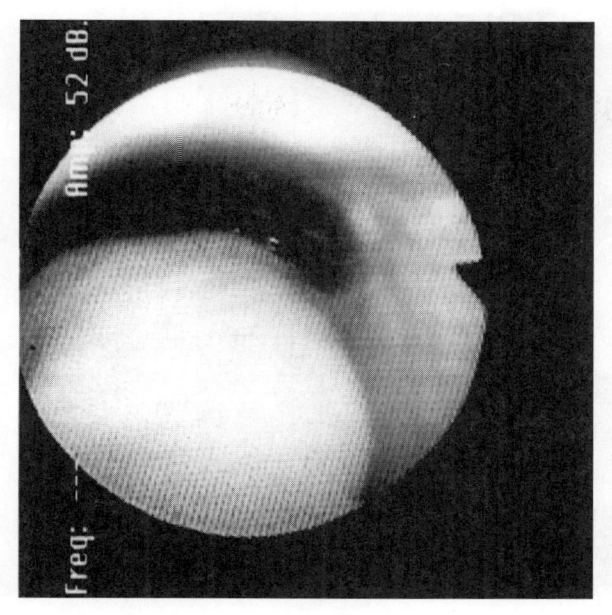

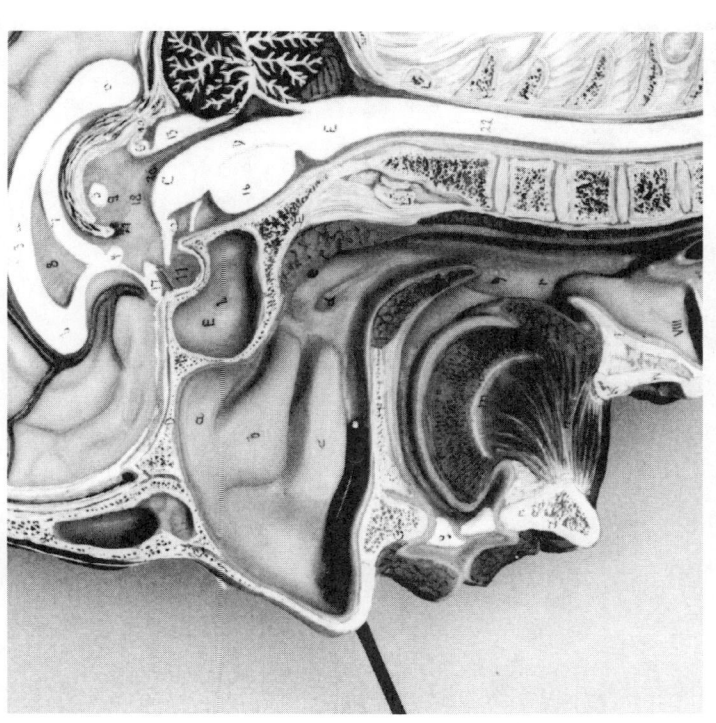

Figure 4–7. Views from insertion through the inferior nasal meatus (*continued*)

65

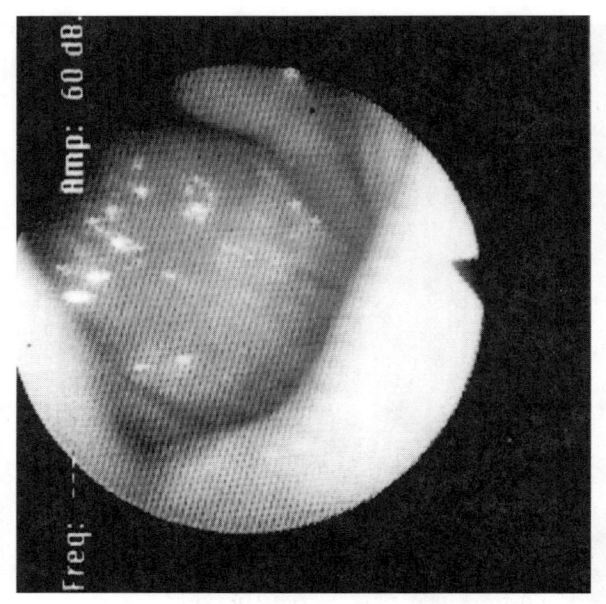

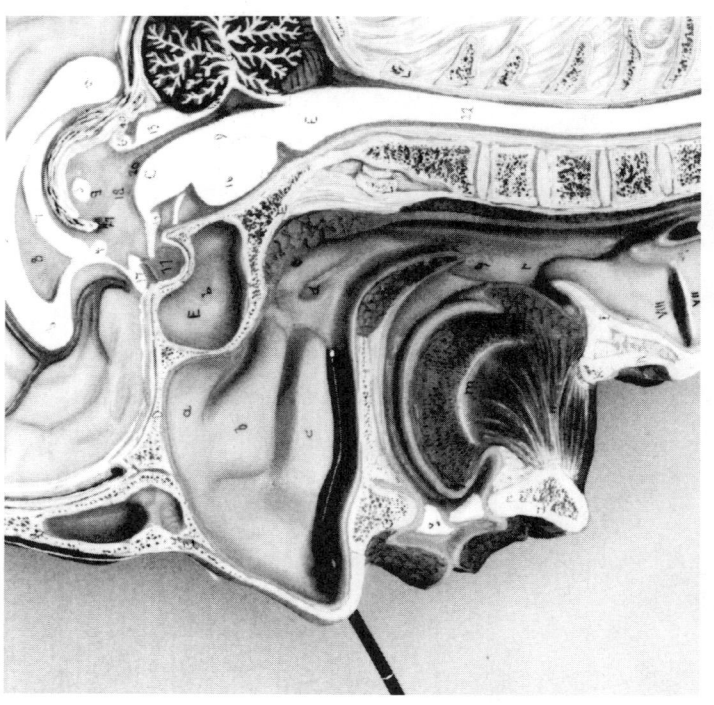

Figure 4–7. Views from insertion through the inferior nasal meatus *(continued)*

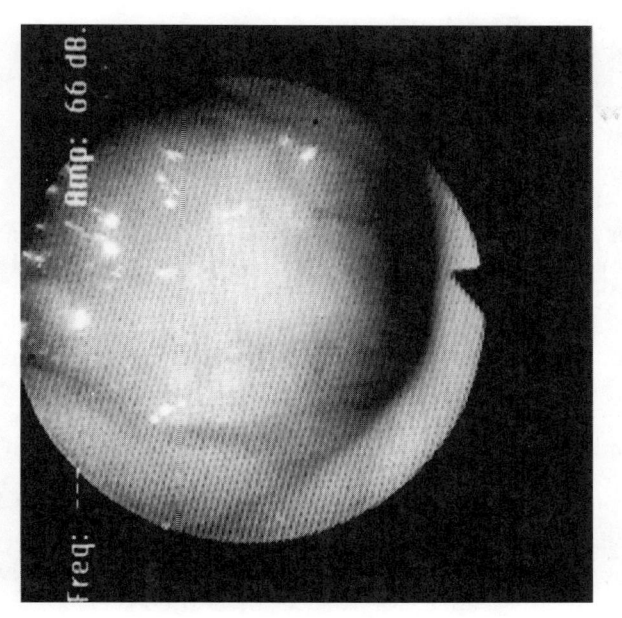

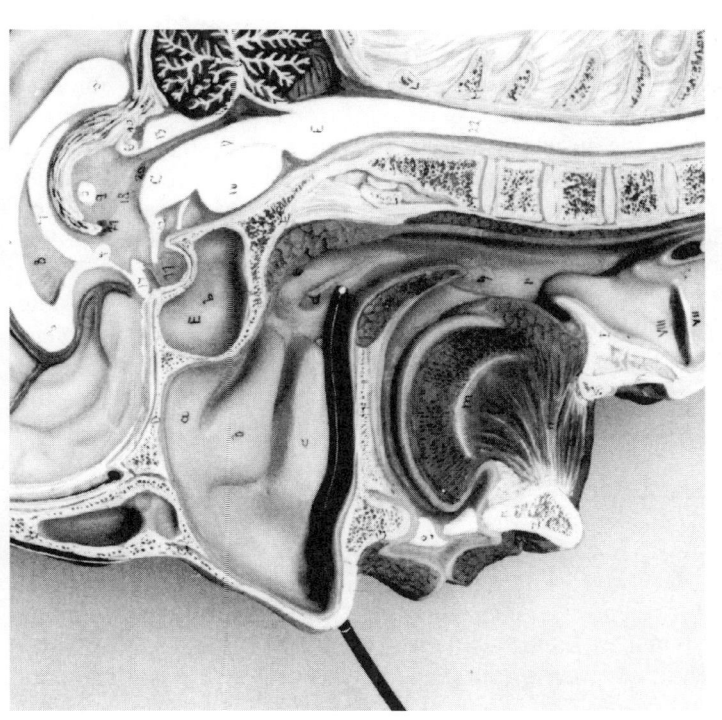

Figure 4–7. Views from insertion through the inferior nasal meatus *(continued)*

examiner may consider completely withdrawing the scope and, after desired anesthetization and vasoconstriction, **repeat the attempt through the opposite nostril.**

3. Scope Positioning After Insertion

After successfully advancing the scope beyond the nasal meatus, the **posterior pharyngeal wall** or **adenoid pad** will usually come into view. The examiner should then stop forward advancement of the scope and adjust the tip, usually by rotating the scope and rocking the scope tip downward to view the velopharyngeal port. Further adjustment of the scope either by advancing, retracting, rotating, or bending the tip should then be performed to achieve the optimal view of the velopharyngeal port during speech (Figure 4–8).

Throughout the scope insertion process and while further adjustments are made, the examiner should simultaneously be instructing the patient to produce the desired speech sample. This is particularly important in children and in anxious adults. By keeping the anxious patient actively involved, there is greater control by the examiner and greater potential for longer tolerance by the patient. In patients who are not anxious, it is sometimes very useful to pause and explain to the patient the structures that are visible as the scope is adjusted. However, the procedure should move along at a comfortable, yet steady, pace so that the **endoscope need be left in place no longer than necessary** to acquire the information needed.

If the scope was successfully inserted through the middle nasal meatus, it may be possible to view the entire velopharyngeal area in a single view. Frequently, however, the scope must be positioned to view one side, then the other, as the patient repeats the desired speech sample.

4. Speech Sample

Careful consideration should be given to the speech sample used. When hypernasality is present and velopharyngeal insufficiency is suspected, the speech samples should be designed to **include all oral samples, samples with multiple nasal consonants,** and **mixed oral and nasal samples** (Table 4–1). The length of each sample should be controlled

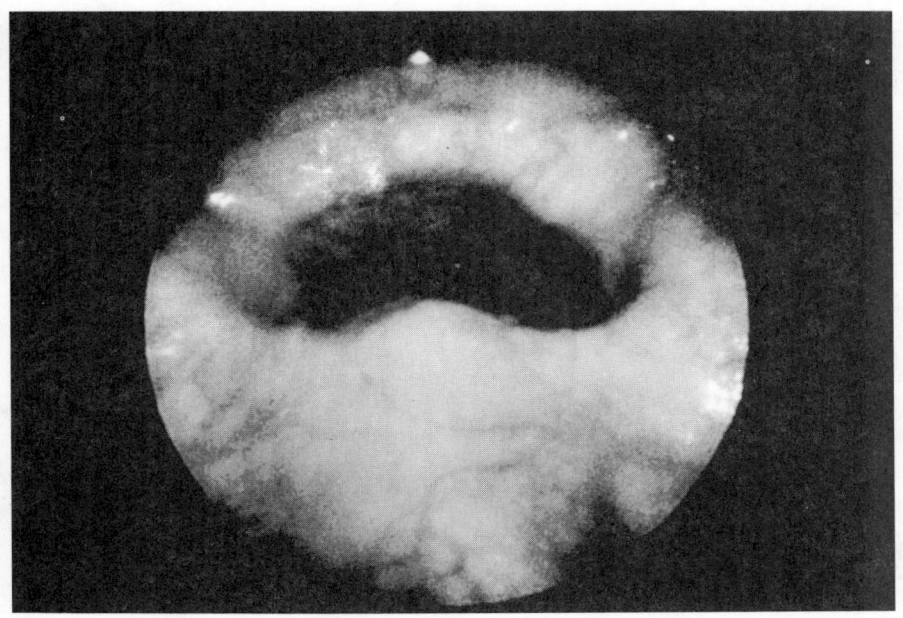

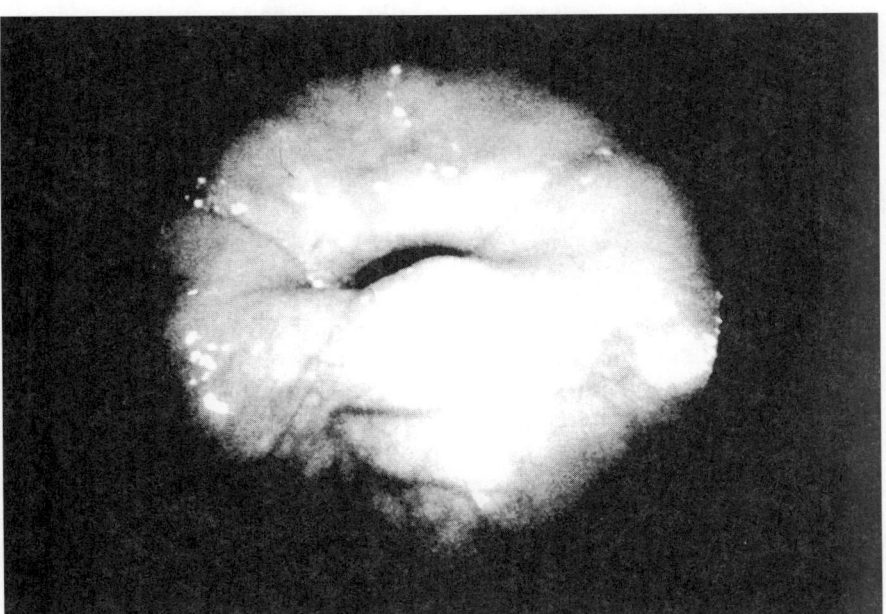

Figure 4–8. An optimal view of a velopharyngeal port during nasal sound production (**top**) and vowel production (**bottom**).

Table 4–1. Examples of speech stimuli used during velopharyngeal endoscopy

High Pressure Stimuli	Low Pressure Stimuli
Sustained oral consonants: [S] [s]	Sustained vowels [ɑ] [u] [i]
Repeated syllables [pɑ] [tɑ] [kɑ]	Repeated syllables [lɑ] [wɑ]
Ride the bus.	You are well.
Go to school.	We were away.
Chop the wood.	Why were you away.
Did Dad do it?	You were away all year.
She wears blue shoes.	Roll a yellow wheel here.

Nasal Stimuli	Mixed Stimuli
Sustained [m]	Repetition of syllables [pɑmɑ]
Repetition of syllables [ma] [na]	Counting from 1 to 10.
Mama made some lemon jam.	Come to my house tonight for ice
Ten men came in when Jane rang.	cream cake.
	Conversational speech.

as well, beginning with brief sustained continuant consonants, moving to short multisyllabic phrases, and proceeding to longer more complex sentences.

a. **All oral samples**. Samples that are devoid of nasal consonants are important to use with patients who are suspected of having velopharyngeal insufficiency and hypernasal speech. All oral samples enable the clinician to observe how the patient moves the velopharyngeal structures when continuous velopharyngeal closure is required for optimal speech production. **Inability to achieve closure** or **failure to maintain closure** may, therefore, be identified. Oral stimuli may be classified as high pressure or low pressure.

(1) **High pressure oral stimuli** contain oral consonants requiring a rapid increase in intraoral air pressure such as sibilants, fricatives, and affricates. High pressure stimuli are useful for demonstrating velopharyngeal function when a maximally tight velopharyngeal seal is necessary. This is particularly important for some patients who achieve adequate closure for low pressure sounds like vowels and who, therefore, have relatively little hypernasality, but who do exhibit audible nasal emission of air.

(2) **Low pressure oral stimuli** contain oral consonants that do not require intraoral air pressure such as glides and liquids. Low pressure oral stimuli permit observation of velopharyngeal function when a maximally tight velopharyngeal seal is not required for normal oral production. Because intraoral air pressure is not necessary during these samples, audible nasal emission will not occur. Normal production of these samples does require adequate velopharyngeal closure, however, in order to avoid hypernasal resonance.

b. **All nasal samples.** Patients with hyponasality require assessment of velopharyngeal opening for nasal consonant production. These patients are frequently those who have undergone secondary surgery (usually pharyngeal flap surgery) to improve velopharyngeal insufficiency. Some of those patients will have difficulty achieving adequate velopharyngeal opening for nasal sound production as well as for nasal respiration.

Speech stimuli that include a high incidence of nasal consonants provide a means for assessing velopharyngeal opening gestures during endoscopy. For patients who have received **pharyngeal flap surgery**, it is important to have the patient repeat these stimuli while the examiner observes both left and right lateral ports.

c. **Mixed stimuli.** Mixed oral and nasal samples provide an opportunity to observe velopharyngeal function when the patient is required to achieve rapid shifts from velopharyngeal opening to velopharyngeal closure. These stimuli place requirements on the patient that are most like **conversational speech**.

d. **Repeated samples**. Multiple repetition of speech stimuli is advisable. Some patients are inconsistent in their ability to achieve velopharyngeal closure. Asking the patient repeat the speech stimuli enables the clinician to assess **consistency of performance**.

B. Velopharyngeal Videoendoscopy—Oral Approach

Oral endoscopy for velopharyngeal evaluation is performed by having the patient sit upright in a comfortable chair (Figure 4–9).

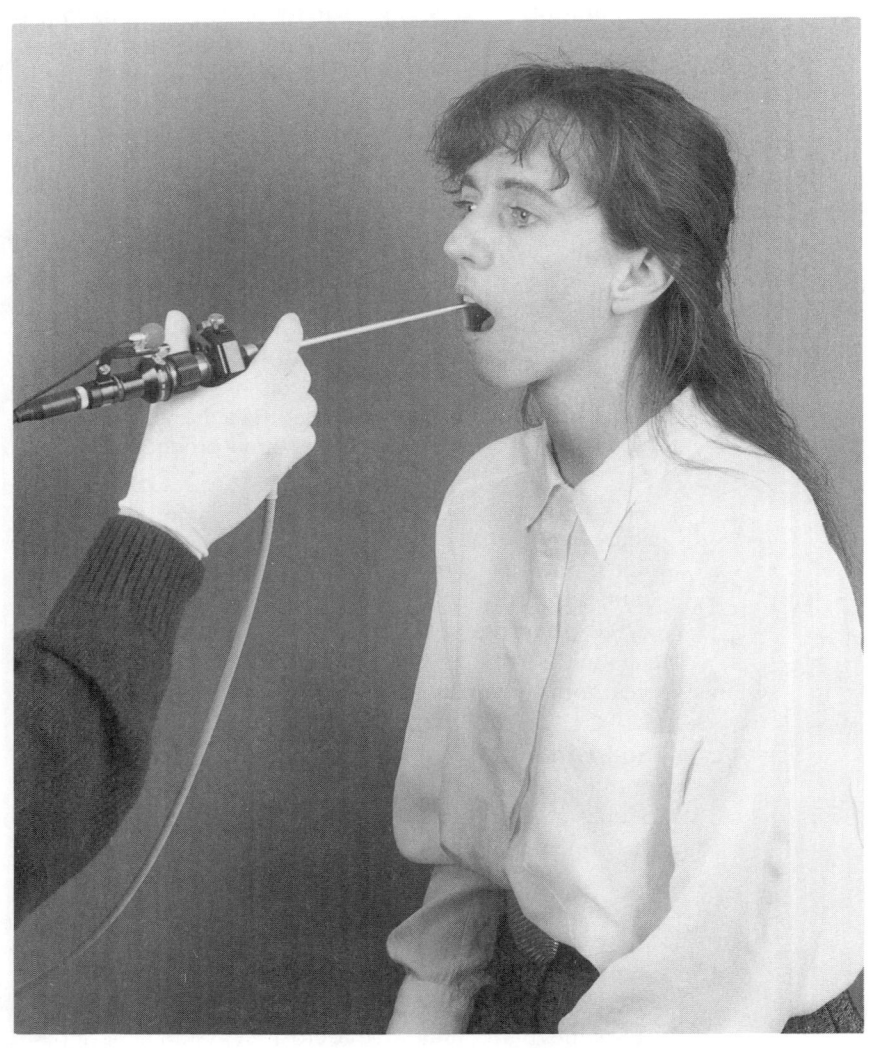

Figure 4–9. Patient positioning for oral endoscopic examination of velopharyngeal closure.

The **use of head rests or restraints is contraindicated for oral endoscopy**. The patient should have the ability to move away from the scope should the gag reflex be triggered. The examiner may be seated or may stand opposite the patient. It is useful to place the video monitor so it is easily viewed by the examiner over the patient's shoulder. This enables the examiner to shift his or her gaze easily from the monitor to the patient's face.

1. Anesthesia

A major advantage of **oral endoscopy** is that it **does not require anesthesia**. Potential for patient discomfort during an oral endoscopic evaluation is limited to stimulation of the **gag reflex**. Some clinicians advocate the use of topical anesthetics to reduce the sensitivity of the gag reflex temporarily in patients who appear to be hypersensitive. Although we generally avoid use of anesthetic application directly to the pharynx, a small dose (two sprays from a hand-held atomizer) may be useful in reducing the gag reflex in hypersensitive patients. The examiner must balance the need for anesthesia against the risk of adverse patient reaction to the typically bitter taste of topical anesthesia. There is also concern that reduced pharyngeal sensitivity may make normal swallowing difficult and may increase the risk of aspiration. There are no data that clearly show that use of oral anesthesia increases the likelihood of laryngospasm.

2. Oral Insertion

Use of oral endoscopy requires careful placement of the endoscope into position in the oropharynx so that the velopharyngeal structures can be viewed while the patient produces the desired speech stimuli. The insertion process is facilitated because the scope's position is easily monitored by the clinician during insertion. Even so, a steady hand and a cooperative patient are necessary. Unless the scope and camera are tripod mounted, the volume of the oral lumen makes potential for movement of the scope within the lumen much greater than during nasal endoscopy. Movements of the tongue during speech further complicate steady positioning of the endo-scope and also increase likelihood of stimulating a gag reflex. **Careful construction of the speech stimuli to minimize tongue movements is extremely important**.

a. **Free camera technique.** In the "free camera" technique, the examiner holds the camera-endoscope apparatus. No tripod is used. The patient is instructed to open his or her mouth comfortably. The end of the endoscope insertion tube is placed on the surface of the tongue and allowed to rest there for 1–2 seconds. This allows the patient to become **accustomed to the feel of the scope** while the lens warms and spontaneously defogs. At this time, the patient may be instructed to produce the desired speech sample (usually [pɑ] or [bɑ] repetitions) so that she or he may become **accustomed to achieving bilabial closure** around the scope.

When these preliminary steps are completed successfully, and appropriate verbal praise is provided the patient, the examiner may slowly move the scope further along the tongue body until the desired view of the velopharyngeal structures is achieved (Figure 4–10).

It may be useful to **anchor the scope between the maxillary central incisors** in some patients. Maxillary stabilization of the rigid endoscope in this fashion may enable the clinician to move the lens successfully into position in the pharynx without the increased risk of evoking a gag reflex that accompanies posterior lingual stimulation. This approach may have the undesirable effect of increasing the difficulty of achieving optimal positioning of the endoscopic lens for observation of velopharyngeal movements due to the angle between the endoscopic lens and the sagittal plane of the velopharyngeal port.

b. **Tripod mounted camera technique.** Fixing the camera/endoscope assembly to a tripod facilitates steady positioning of the scope during insertion and recording of the oral endoscopic procedure. It **requires additional cooperation on the part of the patient**, however, because she or he must slowly advance toward the endoscope, since the position of the endoscope is fixed. The scope may be anchored between the maxillary central incisors or may be stabilized on the superior tongue surface as the patient advances forward until the endoscope lens is positioned in the oropharynx. The patient must then remain quite still after the scope is in position to achieve stable pictures

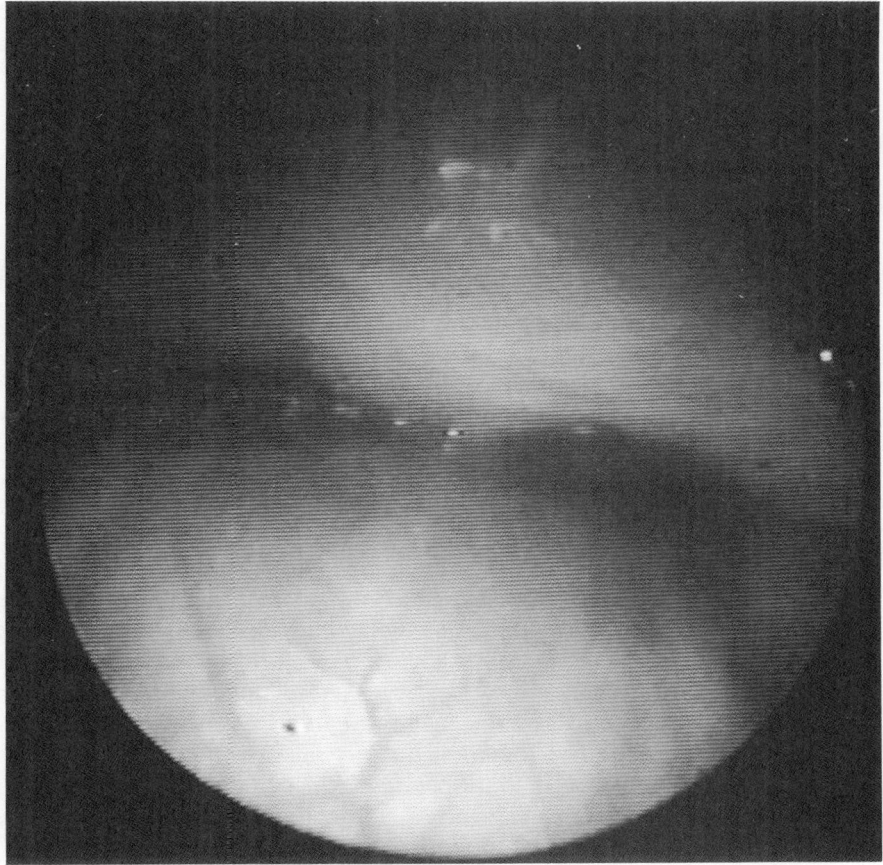

Figure 4–10. Oral videoendoscopic view of the velopharyngeal port during closure. The velum is at the top of the picture; the posterior wall at the bottom.

of velopharyngeal movement and to avoid stimulating a gag reflex.

There is **an additional element of risk for patient discomfort** if the patient moves forward too far or too quickly, allowing the rigid endoscope to contact the posterior pharyngeal wall. Careful patient preparation and clinician monitoring can minimize these risks.

c. **Scope positioning.** The scope should be positioned in the **midline of the oropharynx directly beneath the**

velopharyngeal port. When possible, the scope should be positioned so that all observations can be obtained from a single view. However, rotation of the scope may be accomplished to pan across the width of the velopharyngeal port if necessary.

During oral endoscopic observation of velopharyngeal movements, velar movements appear from the top of the image and extend downward, as closure is approximated, toward the posterior pharyngeal wall. Posterior wall movements appear along the bottom of the image and extend upward toward the velum. Left and right lateral wall movements are oriented as in nasal endoscopic images.

d. **Minimizing gag reflex.** As stated previously, rigid oral endoscopy may stimulate a gag reflex in many patients. To minimize the risk of this unpleasant experience, it is useful to ask the patient to **continue to repeat the speech sample** as the scope is moved posteriorly beyond the faucial arches. This may distract the patient and help reduce sensitivity to the scope. Also, it is not advisable to leave the oral endoscope in place in the oral cavity for more time than is necessary to obtain the information needed. The patient **may need to swallow** as saliva production is increased in response to the presence of the scope. The oral scope should be withdrawn as needed throughout the study to allow the patient to swallow and/or reposition himself for maximum comfort.

3. Speech Sample

As indicated above, the speech sample for oral endoscopic assessment of velopharyngeal function for speech is of particular importance. Tongue movements should be minimized to reduce displacement of the scope within the oropharynx. Therefore, speech **samples that include bilabial consonants and low vowels are preferable**. Examples are provided in Table 4–2.

These repetitions should be performed at a comfortable rate, loudness, and pitch. If the examiner notices that the productions are atypical of usual conversation speech quality, further instruction should be provided until the desired target speech quality is achieved.

Table 4-2. Speech stimuli used for rigid oral endoscopic examination of velopharyngeal function

Nasal Utterances	Oral Utterances	Mixed Oral/Nasal Utterances
Sustained [m]	Sustained [ɑ] [æ]	Repetitions of [bɑmɑ]
Repetitions of [mɑ] [mæ]	Repetitions of [pɑ] [ba]	[pɑmɑ] [bæmæ] [pæmæ]
Hum, Mama, hum.	[pæ] [bæ]	Papa had ham.
	Papa had pop.	Mama had pop.

Multiple repetitions of each utterance are advisable, particularly after removing and reinserting the oral endoscope. This ensures acquisition of representative behaviors from the patient.

II. VELOPHARYNGEAL ASSESSMENT

Endoscopic assessment of velopharyngeal closure requires careful observation of the four major components of velopharyngeal closure during speech production. These include the velum, the right and left lateral pharyngeal walls, and the posterior pharyngeal wall.

A. Velar Movements

The velum is usually the **major component of velopharyngeal closure for speech**. Velar movements normally occur in a posterior-superior direction. Endoscopically, posterior movement appears as an upward excursion of the velum, while superior movement appears as an enlargement of the velum as it nears the nasal endoscope. Velar movements occur relatively high in the velopharyngeal port and are **best viewed by nasal videoendoscopy** (Karnell & Morris, 1985).

B. Lateral Wall Movements

Lateral wall movements appear endoscopically as left-to-right (in the case of the right lateral wall) or right-to-left (in the case of the left lateral wall) displacement of the lateral walls of the velopharynx toward the midline of the velopharyngeal port.

Lateral pharyngeal wall displacement may extend along a broad plane from the level of the velum inferiorly toward the posterior faucial arches. Maximum excursion of the lateral pharyngeal walls usually takes place below the level of the velum and, for this reason, may be examined **best using oral endoscopy** (Karnell & Morris, 1985).

When using **flexible nasal endoscopy, evaluation of lateral wall movement is somewhat complex.** It is useful to move the tip of the scope into the oropharynx so that the base of the tongue and the epiglottis become visible. Then, while the patient produces the desired speech sample, the clinician can slowly withdraw the flexible endoscope back up into the velopharynx while observing lateral wall movement. This manuever makes it possible to identify the extent of lateral wall movement in patients who achieve maximum lateral wall movement below the level of the velum. The extent to which the presence of the flexible endoscope within the velopharyngeal port may influence lateral wall movement has not been determined.

Assessment of the **lateral pharyngeal walls** is of particular importance when contemplating secondary management of **velopharyngeal insufficiency**. Generally, it is important that the patient demonstrate adequate medial movement of the lateral pharyngeal walls if pharyngeal flap surgery is being considered. Pharyngeal flap surgery results in two relatively small lateral ports on either side of the flap (Figure 4–11). Medial movement of the lateral pharyngeal walls may be necessary to close the lateral ports adequately during speech production after pharyngeal flap surgery.

When lateral pharyngeal wall movement is lacking, some clinicians argue that **pharyngeal flap surgery is not indicated** because the patient may fail to close the lateral ports after surgery (Jackson, 1985). In such patients, **sphincter pharyngoplasty** (Hynes, 1950; Orticochea, 1968) may be recommended. Sphincter pharyngoplasty involves raising two lateral flaps, either from the posterior faucial pillars or the lateral pharyngeal walls, and inserting these flaps along the midline of the posterior pharyngeal wall. This usually leaves a relatively small, midline port after surgery which requires posterior movement of the velum for closure during speech (Figure 4–12). However, because the port is considerably smaller than the preoperative port, less velar movement is required. Recently, the importance of inserting the flaps

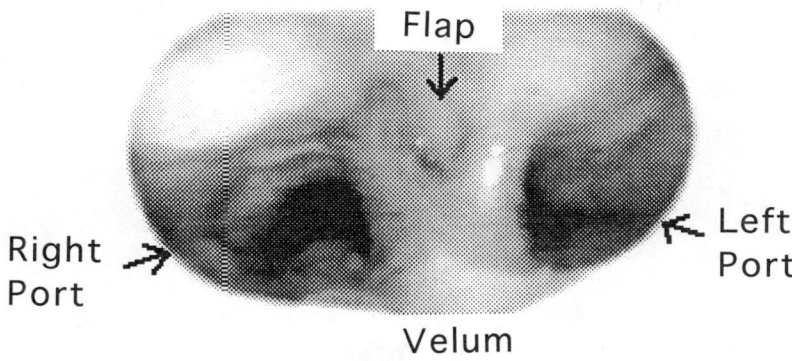

Figure 4–11. A nasal videoendoscopic view of a pharyngeal flap.

at the level of the typical velar movement during speech has been emphasized (Riski et al., 1992).

c. **Posterior Wall Movements**
Assessment of posterior wall movement is important for full understanding of velopharyngeal physiology. It frequently appears as a discrete, anterior bulging of tissue creating the shelf-like appearance of **Passavant's ridge** (Figure 4–13). However, posteror wall displacement may occur over a broad area from the level of the velum to the oropharynx.

Typically, maximum posterior wall movement occurs below the level of maximum velar movement. Therefore, it may be assessed **best by oral endoscopy** or by inserting the **nasal endoscope into the oropharynx** as described for assessment of lateral wall movement.

d. **Velopharyngeal Closure**
The single most important element of endoscopic assessment of velopharyngeal closure is assessment of closure itself. This requires identifying the location, relative size, and timing of any failure to achieve complete velopharyngeal closure when needed for normal oral speech production. Failure may be **severe and consistent**, as in patients with severe velopharyngeal

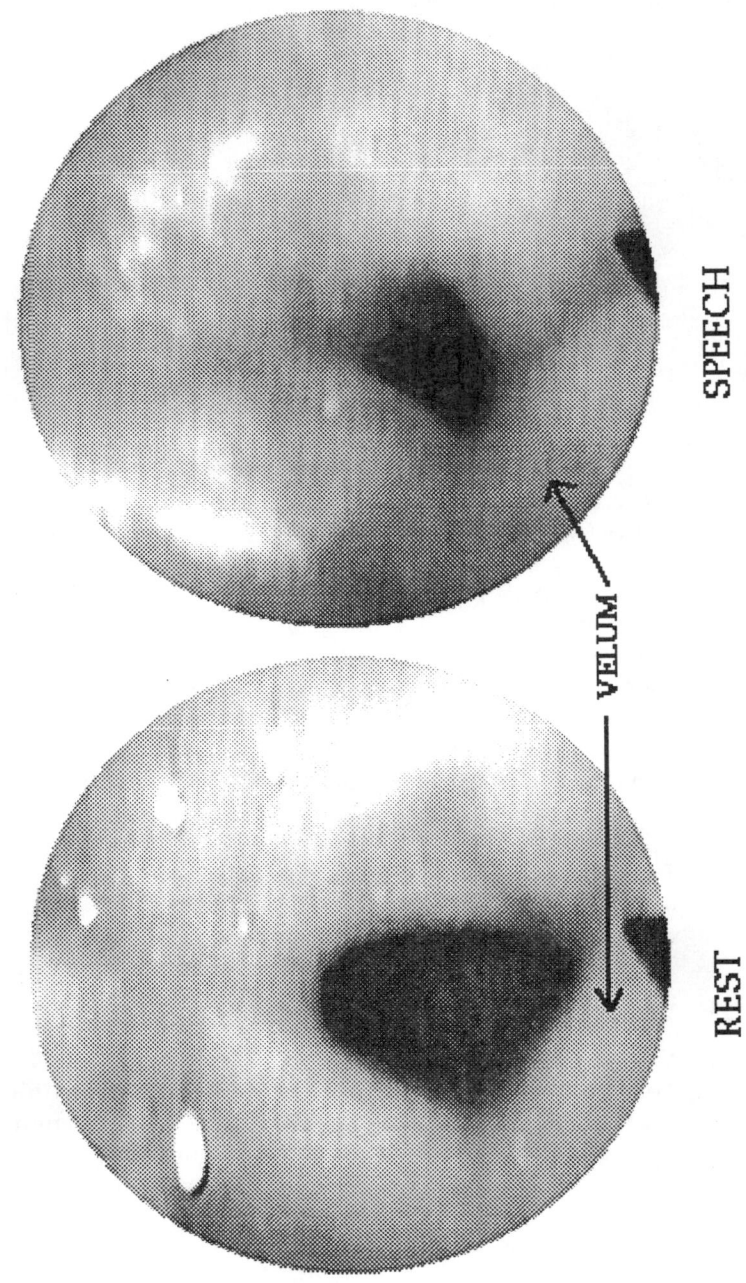

REST

SPEECH

VELUM

Figure 4–12. A nasal videoendoscopic view of a sphincter pharyngoplasty.

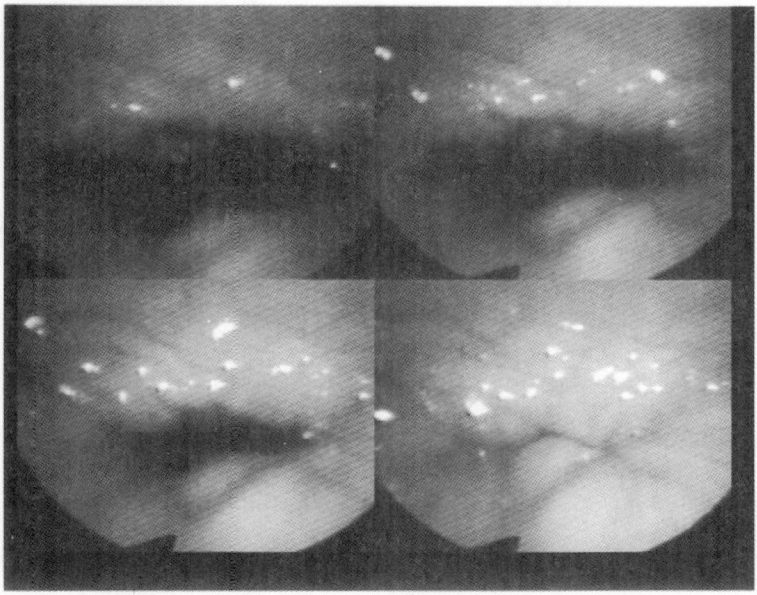

Figure 4–13. A nasal videoendoscopic view of Passavant's ridge. In the series shown here, the posterior wall (**top**) moves anteriorly toward the velum (**bottom**) as the sequence progresses from upper left to lower right.

insufficiency, **or temporary**, as in patients with mild or moderate velopharyngeal insufficiency.

When performing endoscopic assessment of velopharyngeal closure, it is desirable to position the scope so that the **entire velopharyngeal port may be viewed in a single image**. However, this is not always possible, particularly in small adults and children, because the dimensions of the nasopharynx (or oropharynx in the case of oral endoscopy) may be too small to permit adequate separation between the velopharyngeal structures and the endoscopic lens. In such cases, it is necessary to rotate the endoscope slightly in order to pan across the velopharyngeal port as the patient produces the speech stimuli.

1. Location

The location of breaches in velopharyngeal closure are variable from patient to patient. It is, therefore, **particularly** important to determine the location, as well as the size, of any breach in closure when considering management options. Location of the velopharyngeal opening may be characterized as **midline or lateral** and, if lateral, unilateral (specify right or left) or bilateral.

2. Size

Assessment of the relative size of the velopharyngeal gap is also important when management is considered. If **pharyngeal flap surgery** is considered the treatment of choice, it is important that the size of the pharyngeal flap be adequate to occlude the gap but that it not be so wide as to prevent nasal respiration and normal nasal resonance for speech. It has been shown that surgical customizing of pharyngeal flap width is possible, to a limited extent (Shprintzen et al., 1979).

3. Consistency

Patients who exhibit inconsistent velopharyngeal closure for speech are frequently the most difficult to manage. Such patients exhibit ability to achieve adequate velolpharyngeal closure sometimes, but they fail to achieve closure at other times (Morris, 1984). To make matters more difficult, the nature of this inconsistency varies from patient to patient.

For the purpose of this discussion, **two general types of inconsistent velopharyngeal closure** will be considered. The first, and more common, is inconsistency within a given utterance. The second, is inconsistency between utterances.

a. **Within-utterance inconsistency.** Patients who exhibit within-utterance inconsistency may achieve velopharyngeal closure at discrete moments during an utterance but permit velopharyngeal gaps at other moments. Some of these patients have difficulty with only one or two phonemes (usually [s] and [z]) and may be described, therefore, as having **phoneme specific velopharyngeal insufficiency**. These cases usually involve sibilant production and represent a failure to learn velopharyngeal closure during production of the phonemes in question. Appropriate treatment, therefore, is speech therapy.

Another group of patients with within-utterance inconsistency are those whose breaches in velopharyngeal closure appear to be related to the **complex interaction between force of closure, velar elevation, oral speech articulator movement and speech aerodynamics**. The details of how the individual members of this group manifest inconsistent velopharyngeal closure vary depending on the interaction of these variables.

For example, if velopharyngeal closure is achievable, but force of closure is inadequate, momentary breaches of closure may occur with increases in intraoral air pressure associated with pressure consonants. Perceptually, these patients exhibit **audible nasal emission of air** during pressure consonant productions while having relatively little hypernasal resonance.

If the patient is capable of achieving complete closure only when the velum is at the point of maximum excursion, breaches in closure may occur when the patient produces low vowels such as [ɑ], [ɛ], [æ], and so on. Such vowel productions are frequently associated with **lower velar positions**. When the velum lowers for these sounds from maximum velar height, associated with a high vowel or pressure consonant, momentary breaches in closure may occur, resulting in acoustic resonance in the nasal cavities perceived as **hypernasality** (Figure 4–14). Audible nasal emission of air may or may not occur in these patients depending on the timing on intraoral air pressure variations and the timing of the shifts in velar position.

Another group of patients who exhibit within-utterance inconsistency are those who appear to **relax their velopharyngeal mechanism with reduced linguistic stress**. These individuals tend to permit velopharyngeal opening during unstressed syllables but achieve closure during stressed syllables.

b. **Between-utterance inconsistency.** Patients who exhibit between-utterance inconsistency are those who **achieve adequate and appropriate closure** for a given utterance produced at **time one, but fail to achieve closure** for the same utterance **at time two** (Figure 4–15). These

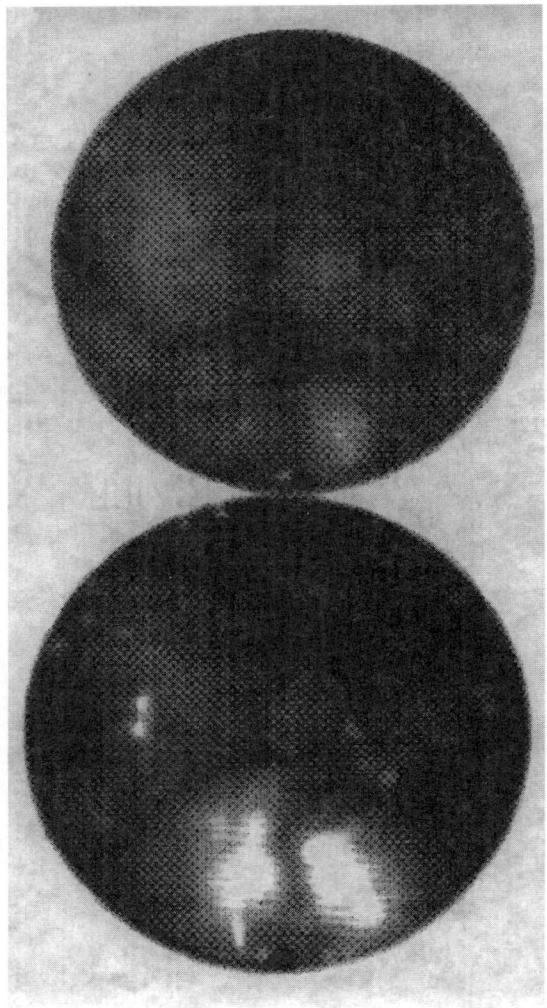

Figure 4-14. Velopharyngeal incompetence during vowel production (**top**) followed by adequate closure during the subsequent consonant (**bottom**).

patients appear to perform better during the structured, controlled environment of the speech evaluation than during unstructured conversational activities.

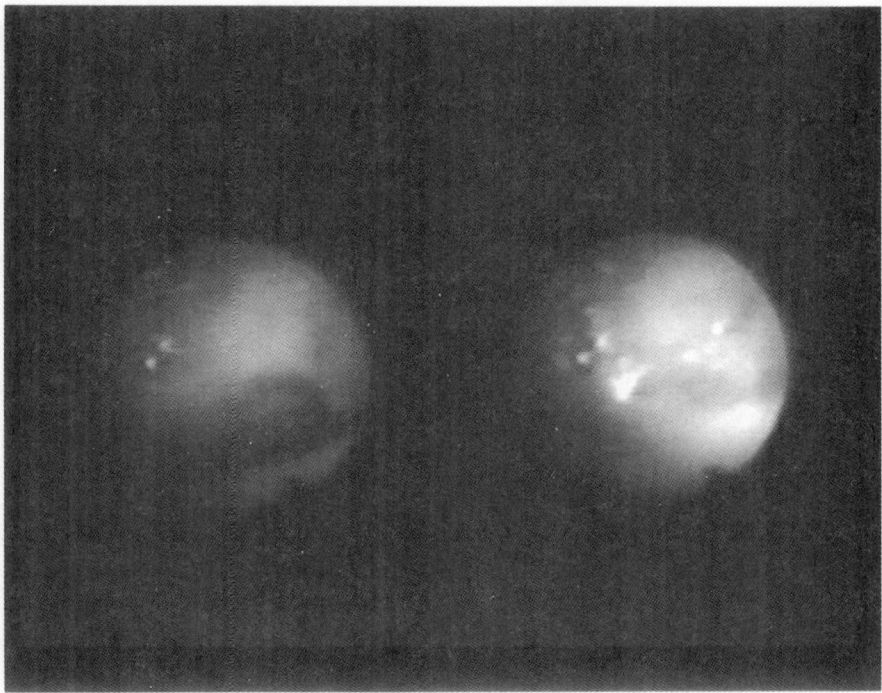

Figure 4–15. Between-utterance inconsistent closure. Velopharyngeal opening observed during an initial production of "Did Dad do it?" followed by closure during a second production of the same sentence.

E. Ratings and Measurements

Endoscopic assessment of velopharyngeal function for speech involves careful inspection and description of the velopharyngeal structures and closure. Descriptions may be narrative or may include ratings or measurements (Golding-Kushner et al., 1990; Karnell et al., 1983) of the various components of velopharyngeal closure.

1. Ratings

The **most detailed system** for rating velopharyngeal movements is described by Golding-Kushner et al. (1990). A complete description of that system is beyond the scope of this discussion. Brifely, each component of velopharyngeal closure is related as a proportion of maximum potential velopharyngeal movement or closure. For example, the full range of potential velar movements extends from the posterior edge of the midline of the velum when at rest to the point on the posterior pharyngeal wall where that same point on the velum would make contact during closure. If one can imagine the full range of this potential movement as extending from 0% movement at rest to 100% movement at the point of posterior wall contact, actual observed movement can be rated as some ratio between these two extremes. A velum that moves only halfway across the potential range of movement would be rated as achieving 50% movement (Figure 4–16). The other components of closure, the posterior wall and lateral walls, are rated in a similar fashion.

The size of the velopharyngeal port may also be rated as some ratio of complete closure. The Golding-Kushner et al. system suggests rating closure from 0–100%, where 0% relates to status at rest or during nasal respiration, and 100% reflects complete closure. Another approach, and one that might seem more physiologic to some, would be to rate

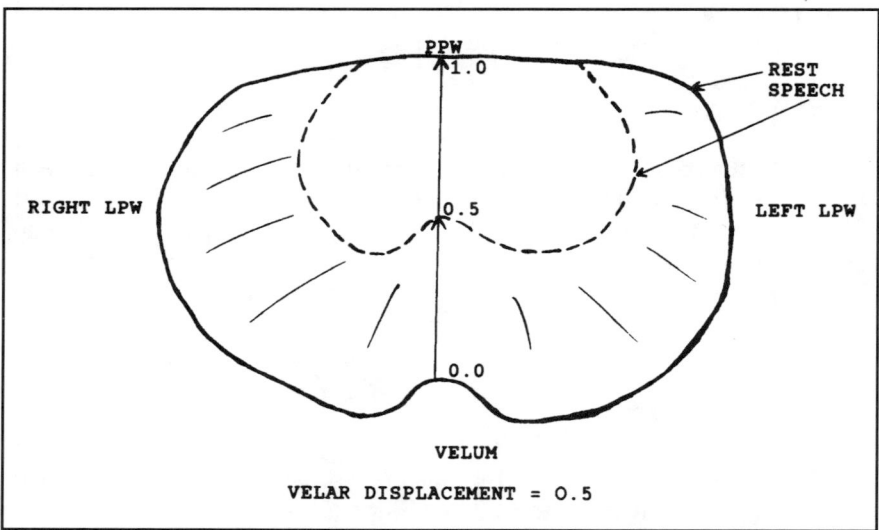

Figure 4–16. Rating system for velar movement (from Golding-Kushner et al., 1990).

velopharyngeal opening rather than velopharyngeal closure. Rating opening would reverse the scale so that the status at rest or during nasal respiration would reflect 100% opening, and the status during complete closure would be rated as 0% opening (Figure 4–17). This approach reflects the inverse relationship between velopharyngeal movements and the size of velopharyngeal opening.

2. Measurements

It is possible to further objectify the rating system described above by making **actual measurements from the video-endoscopic images**. Such measurements could be obtained from the video monitor (Karnell, Linville, & Edwards, 1988) or by using digital image processing techniques. Because the measurements are ratios, the actual units are arbitrary. For

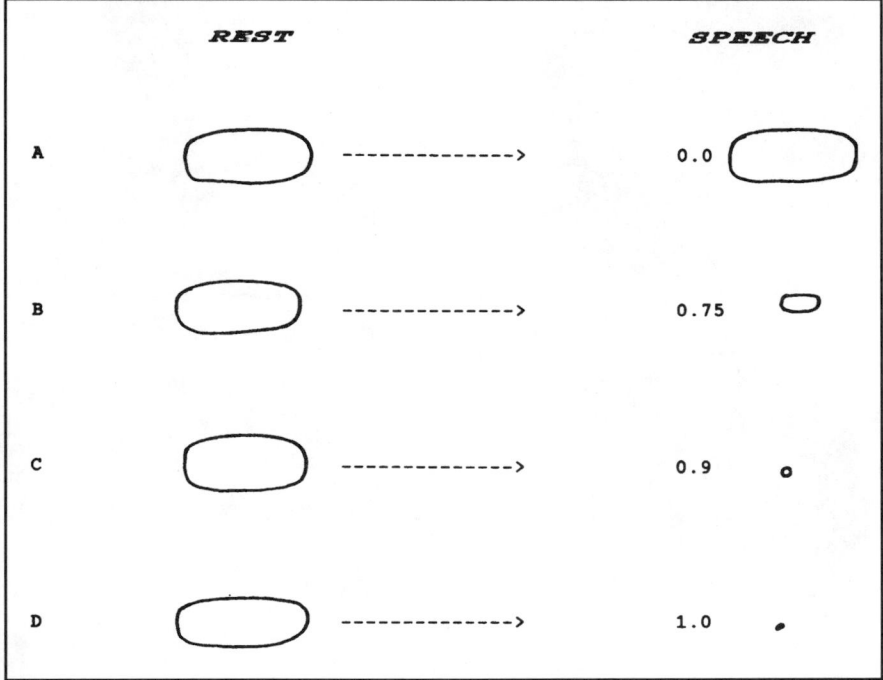

Figure 4–17. Rating system for velopharyngeal closure (from Golding-Kushner et al., 1990).

example, measurements of the distance between the nasal surface of the soft palate and the posterior pharyngeal wall at rest could be made in pixels, using digital image processing. The same measurement could be made after excursion of the soft palate toward the posterior wall (Figure 4–18). The ratio of movement would be calculated as follows:

$$\frac{\text{Measurement (in pixels) after movement}}{\text{Measurement (in pixels) before movment}} \times 100 = \% \text{ movement}$$

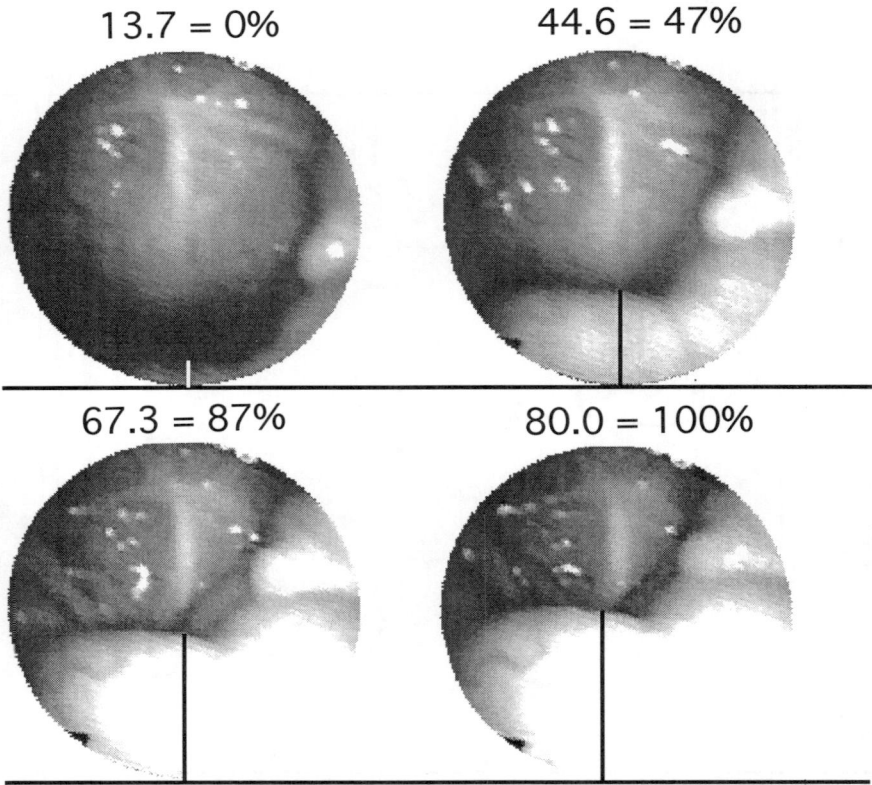

13.7 = 0%   44.6 = 47%

67.3 = 87%   80.0 = 100%

Figure 4–18. Measurement system for velar movement (see text for detailed explanation).

Precautions should be taken, however, to ensure that **no change in the relative position of the endoscope** within the nasopharynx (or oropharynx if oral endoscopy is used) occurs when denominator and numerator measurements are made.

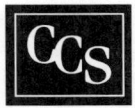

CHAPTER

5

Laryngeal Videoendoscopy

There is considerable overlap between procedures employed for video-endoscopic examination of the larynx and procedures for examination of the velopharynx. In this chapter, special consideraton will be given to details that are specific to the laryngeal examination.

I. PROCEDURES

Like velopharyngeal videoendoscopy, laryngeal videoendoscopy can be performed either by nasal or oral approaches. Consideration of both approaches is provided below.

A. Laryngeal Videoendoscopy—Nasal Approach

Nasal videoendoscopy for laryngeal evaluation is identical to that for velopharyngeal endoscopy with regard to insertion through the nasal cavity. It differs, however, in that the flexible endoscope is passed through the **velopharyngeal port** into the oropharynx and hypopharynx. Therefore, **special considerations regarding anesthesia and insertion technique must be addressed**.

1. Anesthesia

Anesthesia for nasal endoscopy applied to laryngeal evaluation is similar to that described for velopharyngeal evaluation. Some clinicians use application of orally applied topical anesthetic to reduce pharyngeal sensitivity to the flexible endoscope. This is performed along with nasal anesthesia. In the author's experience, application of oral anesthesia is rarely necessary for flexible nasal videoendoscopy.

The majority of successful nasal endoscopic examinations of the larynx are performed on adult patients. Adults increased tendency for cooperation, decreased sensitivity to the scope, and larger nasal lumen usually result in reduced need for anesthesia. As stated previously, **some clinicians feel that nasal anesthesia in adult patients is completely unnecessary** (Karnell et al., 1992).

2. Nasal Insertion

Nasal insertion of the flexible endoscope for laryngeal endoscopy/stroboscopy is performed in the same manner as for evaluation of velopharyngeal closure. **Insertion through the middle nasal meatus is preferable**, because the flexible insertion tube is more likely to be suspended above the soft palate and, after insertion through the velopharyngeal lumen, along the posterior pharyngeal wall rather than along the superior surface of the velum. This minimizes the complicating effects velar elevation may have on scope position during the study.

In most patients, it is necessary to insert the scope through only one nasal passage rather than both. **The preferred side is usually the one with the larger lumen**. Lumen size frequently can be inferred from patient reports about nasal obstruction and/or clinical observation of differences in perceived air flow between the right and left nasal passages as the patient breathes through the nose. The patient should be asked if he or she perceives difficulty breathing comfortably through the nose and whether there is any difference between nostrils. If no difference is reported, the clinician should instruct the patient to breathe nasally with the mouth closed while the clinician gently occludes the anterior nares on one side and then the other. Any significant difference in nasal airflow may be perceived using this maneuver.

Differences in nasal lumen size may also be assessed by inserting the flexible endoscope into the nasal vestibule and **observing the anterior size and configuration of the nasal turbinates and septum**. An open anterior nares does not imply an adequate lumen along the entire length of the nostril, however. Middle or posterior nasal lumen constrictions may not be visible from the anterior nasal lumen.

For **a few patients, the view of the larynx may differ significantly** when the scope is placed in one nostril compared to the other. The difference could be very important if the view of the true vocal folds is obscured due to lateral positioning of the endoscope in the pharynx or laryngeal deviation from midline. The clinician should be prepared to remove the endoscope in such cases, apply anesthesia to the opposite nostril, and reinsert.

Advancing the flexible nasal endoscope for laryngeal evaluation must be performed with **a special degree of caution**. Because the tip of the endoscope will be positioned within areas that are sensitive to tactile stimulation, it is important to avoid touching pharyngeal and laryngeal structures with the endoscope during the insertion and evaluation procedures. The open pharyngeal lumen usually makes this task relatively easy.

From the position of the flexible endoscope in the nasopharynx, the scope must first be advanced through the **velopharyngeal port**. This is facilitated by asking the patient to close his or her mouth and breath through the nose; this maneuver opens the velopharyngeal port. The scope should then be gently advanced to a position just posterior to the tongue dorsum in the oropharynx above the level of the superior surface of the epiglottis.

3. Scope Positioning

It is usually advisable to position the endoscope to **approximate the midline of the lumen** while in the oropharynx. From this perspective, the clinician may observe the surfaces of the tongue dorsum, the valeculae, the epiglottis, and the pharyngeal walls with the interior laryngeal structures below in the hypopharynx. Any abnormal or unusual observations such as focal swelling, polyps, or tumors affecting these structures should be carefully visualized for later discussion with the patient and/or the referring health care professional.

The flexible endoscope should **remain above the superior aspect of the epiglottis except when the patient is actively phonating**. Positioning the endoscope in the airway behind the epiglottis or within the laryngeal vestibule frequently results in reflexive coughing or gagging if the patient spontaneously swallows or speaks. Insertion of the endoscope into the **laryngeal vestibule** is possible, however, for close observation of the vocal folds during quiet respiration. This specialized maneuver will be described in detail later.

With the endoscope positioned in the oropharynx above the level of the epiglottis, it is useful to ask the patient to **whistle** a simple tune ("Happy Birthday," for example) while the scope is positioned in the oropharynx so that **gross arytenoid movement** may be assessed. Whistling usually involves laryngeal valving of the airstream, resulting in rapid adduction/abduction maneuvers of the arytenoids. If a unilateral paresis or paralysis is present, it is usually clearly observed. If the patient cannot or will not whistle, simple repetitions of the syllable [hi] will have a similar effect.

Observation of the **ventricular and true vocal folds** should proceed first by having the patient produce a sustained [i] or [u] vowel. These vowels require anterior displacement of the tongue dorsum and pharyngeal dilation, increasing the pharyngeal lumen and facilitating endoscope advancement and positioning. The patient should be instructed to sustain these sounds for as long as is comfortably possible. Measurement of maximum phonation time prior to insertion of the endoscope gives the clinician a good idea about what to expect from the patient. Even so, it is wise to ask the patient to perform sustained phonation for as long as possible with the scope positioned in the oropharynx before advancement into the laryngeal vestibule is attempted.

The clinician should carefully advance the scope into the laryngeal vestibule while the patient is phonating or after instructing the patient not to swallow, again taking care to avoid contact with any laryngeal structures. The flexible insertion tube tip position may be controlled in a precise manner by manipulating the control arm, which changes the angle of the tip of the scope, and by gently rotating the insertion tube, which moves the tip laterally through the pharynx. In this manner, the clinician should be able to advance and position the scope to a point just above the ventricular vocal folds such that, assuming a relatively normal laryngeal mechanism, **the entire length of the true vocal folds is visible** (Figure 5–1). At this point, observations about the color and texture of the vocal fold mucosa are usually possible.

If the patient is phonating, the stroboscopic light may be engaged so that the **vibratory characteristics of the vocal folds** may be assessed. Observations may be made regarding the extent and symmetry of the **amplitude** of the vibrations, **phase symmetry**, **glottal closure**, presence of **nonvibrating segments**, and presence and character of the **mucosal wave**. A data base system for storing, retrieving, and reporting observations of videostroboscopic evaluations will be described later.

The patient should be instructed to produce sustained vowel sounds at a "comfortable" pitch and loudness, without vibrato, while maintaining a constant pitch in order to facilitate examination of vocal fold vibration that is similar to that which occurs during **conversation**. If the patient produces a tone that is substantially different from conversational voice, the clinician may ask the patient to count to three and to sustain the [i] sound at the end of the word "three." This usually induces a closer approximation of the patient's conversational pitch and loudness.

After sampling sustained voice at conversational pitch and loudness, the patient should be instructed to increase pitch gradually from conversational pitch to his or her highest sustainable voice. The patient should be instructed to sustain the high pitch again for several seconds to allow for adequate observation time. Vocal intensity at maximum pitch should also be varied from soft to loud. Observation of vocal fold vibratory activity during these maneuvers may reveal **small mucosal or submucosal lesions** not visible during habitual pitch and loudness (Figure 5–2). These lesions may be more

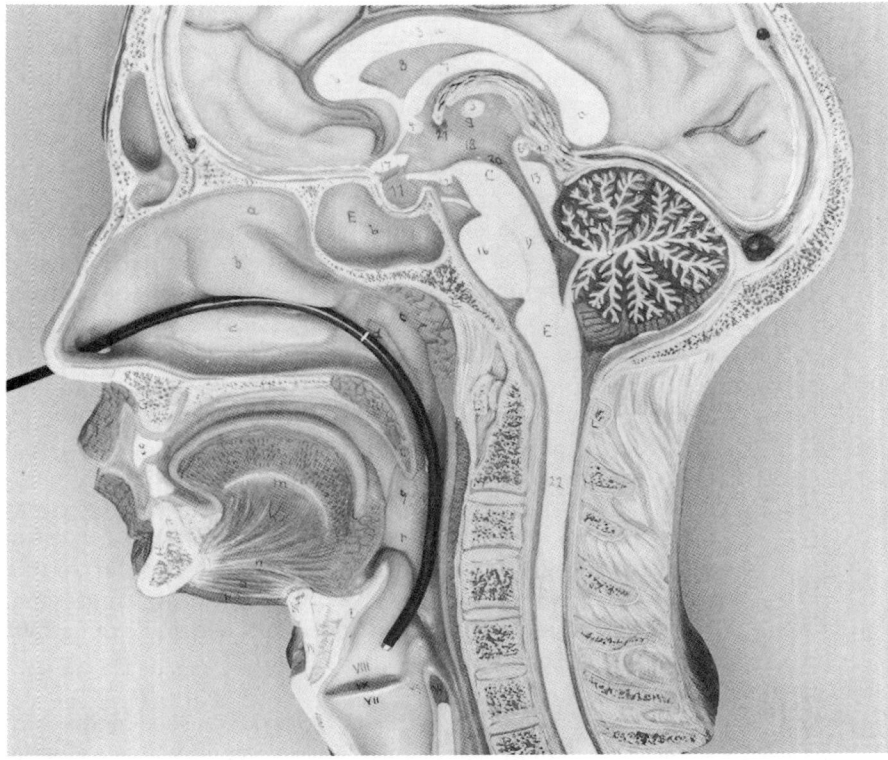

Figure 5-1. Position of the flexible endoscope for close inspection of the vocal folds.

apparent when the vocal folds are stretched as is necessary for high pitch phonation.

If the patient is a **singer**, it is important to be prepared to sample singing as well as non-singing vocal behavior. Trained singers require a period of vocal warm-up exercises before they can be expected to produce their optimal vocal performance, so adequate time for warm-up exercises should be allowed just prior to the stroboscopic evaluation. Also, the singer will likely perform best if allowed to stand during the evaluation.

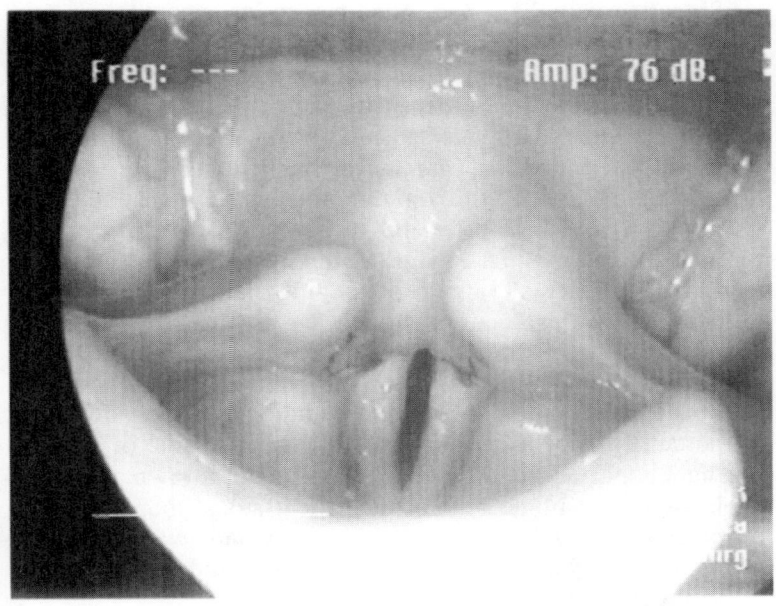

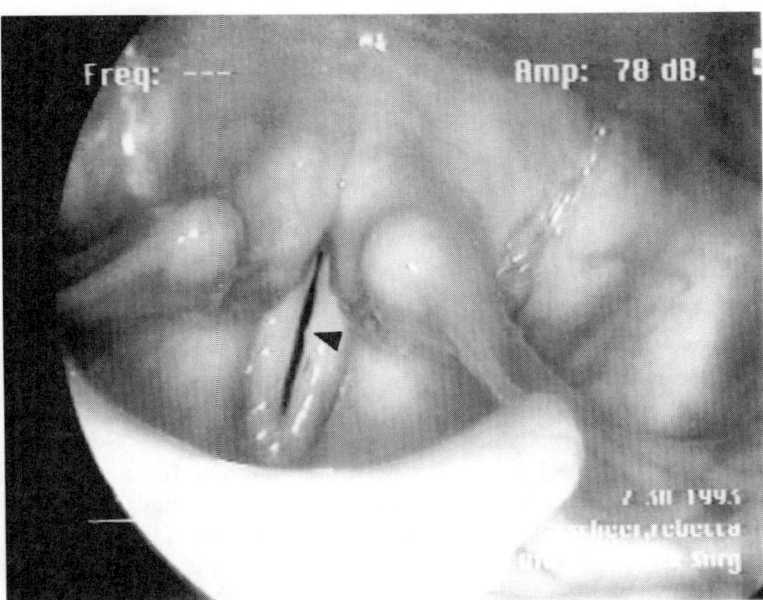

Figure 5-2. A small nodule visible during sustained high pitch phonation (see arrow in bottom photo) that was less visible during sustained habitual pitch (**top**).

Singers usually have very good perceptions about which part of their vocal range is being affected by whatever pathological condition they may be experiencing. Special attention should, obviously, be given to examining that part of the singer's range. This is most commonly accomplished by asking the singer to vary his or her singing voice from a lower pitch upward through the problem pitch area and back down. It may also be useful to have the singer begin at a high pitch and sing downward through the problem range. Finally, an actual sample of singing should be elicited to complete the evaluation.

The clinician should be **cognizant of the patient's status at all times** during the stroboscopic examination. It is important to know how long the patient is capable of sustaining phonation so the scope may be withdrawn from the laryngeal vestibule before the patient stops phonating. The patient may then be permitted to inhale and swallow as well as report any concerns or discomforts to the clinician prior to proceeding with another phonation.

B. Laryngeal Endoscopy—Oral Approach

Oral endoscopy is frequently preferred over nasal endoscopy for the purposes of laryngeal observation. The benefits of **superior image resolution, color representation, and magnification** outweigh the weaknesses of oral articulatory obstruction when the purpose of the study is to view the larynx during respiration or during sustained vowel production. Yanagisawa and Yanagisawa (1993) performed both rigid oral and flexible nasal endoscopy on 120 patients with complaint of hoarseness. Image quality of each study was rated, using a 4-point scale, regarding ability to visualize the vocal folds and ability to observe vibratory pattern. The image quality provided by the rigid oral approach was judged superior 84% of the time, equal 8%, and inferior 7%. Sodersten and Lindestad (1992) utilized a similar method for a different purpose. Five judges rated glottal configuration and degree of closure in 15 normal subjects who underwent both telescopic and flexible endoscopy. A higher degree of incomplete closure was noted from the telescopic examinations. The authors suggested this was due to the unnatural position assumed by patients during this examination. They did not confirm this, however, by replicating patient positioning used during oral endoscopy when performing flexible endoscopic examinations. Further study is warranted to determine the extent to which patient positioning has important effects on image interpretation.

Procedures for oral endoscopy applied to laryngeal examination are very similar to those for velopharyngeal examination. As stated previously, use of oral anesthesia is unnecessary in most cases.

1. Oral Insertion

As described above, the endoscopes used for oral laryngeal evaluation are considerably different from those used for oral velopharyngeal evaluation. First, they are larger in diameter in order to accommodate greater light carrying capacity. Greater illumination is needed for laryngeal evaluations than for velopharyngeal evaluations because of the larger hypo-pharyngeal area to be illuminated and the greater distance between the scope lens positioned in the oropharynx and the vocal folds. Given the larger diameter of the insertion tube, these scopes may be more challenging for the patient to tolerate. **Oral laryngeal scopes provide a magnified view**. This is important, given the distance between the oropharynx and the vocal folds.

a. **90° technique**. If a 90° rigid endoscope is used, the patient may sit upright as during a laryngeal examination (Figure 5–3). The angle between the oral cavity and the pharynx should approximate 90°. **Tongue anchoring** may or may not be necessary to achieve an adequate view of the entire length of the vocal folds.

b. **70° technique.** If a 70° rigid scope is used for laryngeal videoendoscopy, it will be necessary to approximate a 70° oral cavity/pharynx angle. This may be accomplished in either of two ways. The patient may be instructed to bend the upper body forward from the waist. Then the patient should be instructed to lift his or her chin until the head and oral cavity approximate a 70° angle relative to the pharynx (Figure 5–4). It may be helpful to instruct the patient to place his or her elbows on the thighs near

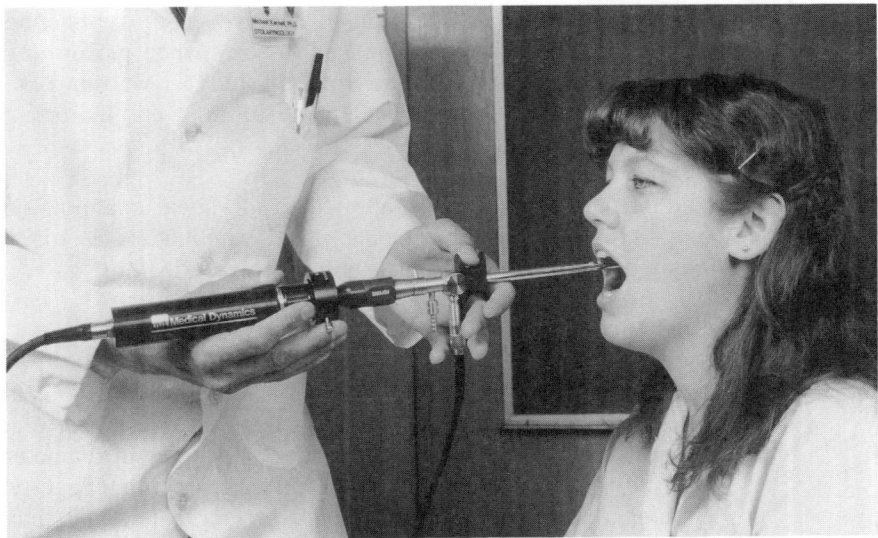

Figure 5–3. During rigid oral endoscopy with a 90° endoscope, the patient is seated in an upright position.

the knees. This position may provide for **better patient stability and comfort** throughout the study. The examiner may choose to be seated or to stand.

An alternative approach to positioning the 70° scope is to have the patient sit upright while rotating his or her chin up and back until the desired angle is achieved. It may be necessary for the examiner to stand in order to position the scope for a proper view with this approach.

For laryngeal evaluation, **the end of the endoscope should be placed on the patient's upper teeth between the central incisors**. This provides a stable maxillary base for the scope above the tongue body. It is sometimes useful and necessary to train the patient to produce the desired, sustained [i] voice sample when the tip of the scope is in this anterior oral cavity position. Patients who spontaneously attempt to avoid lingual contact with the scope may leave the mandible lowered, making an adequate [i] impossible to produce and, therefore, an adequate view impossible to achieve. With the scope placed anteriorly, the patient may be instructed, as

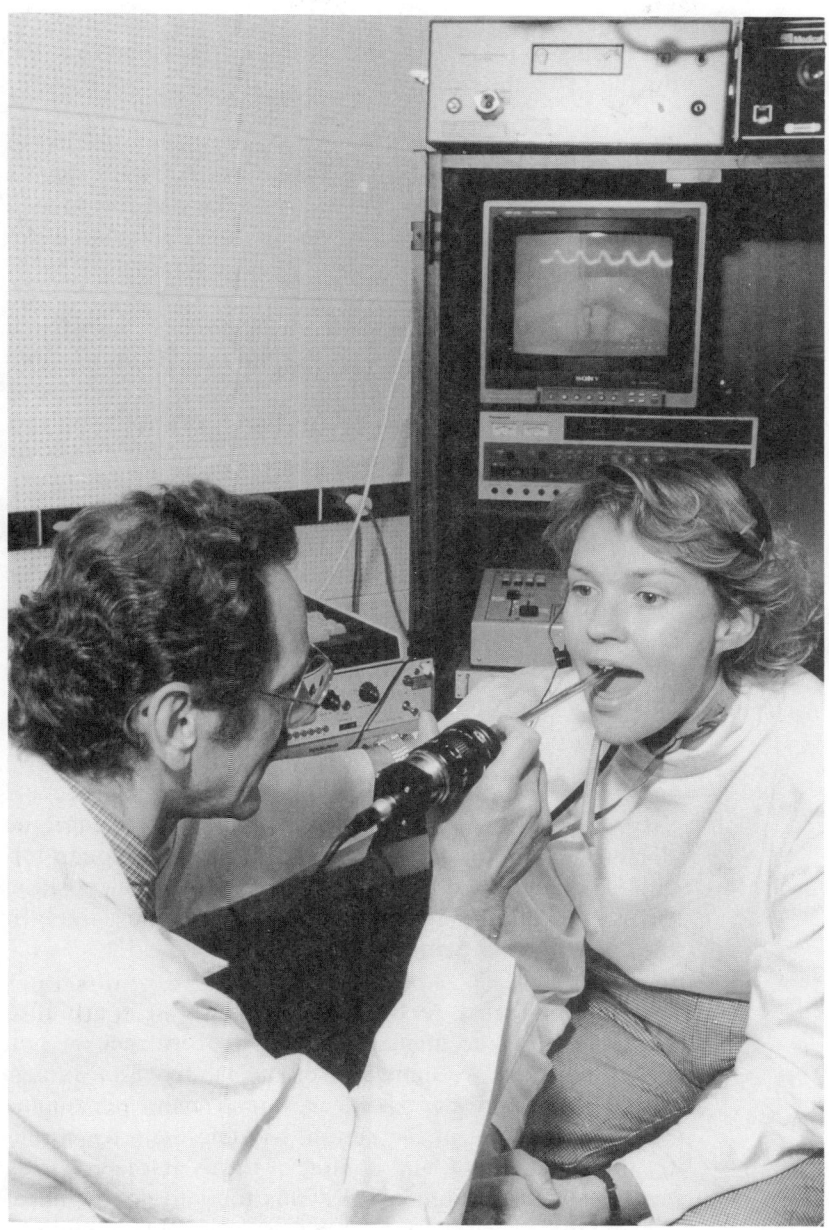

Figure 5–4. The patient is instructed to lean forward during rigid oral endoscopy with a 70° endoscope.

needed, to approximate the desired speech sample without having to tolerate the placement of the scope over the tongue or in the oropharynx.

The voice sample should be adequately long and loud to permit the stroboscopic light source to track the patient's fundamental frequency accurately. **Adequacy of the speech sample** can be monitored by viewing the light source frequency display at this point in the examination.

When it is clear that the patient can produce the desired [i] production, the scope may be moved posteriorly into the **oropharynx**. The patient is instructed to produced additional [i] repetitions while the examiner monitors the view.

In some patients, it is necessary to make small adjustments in scope position after the vocal folds are in view in order to achieve an optimum view. This is sometimes difficult, because the scope can become snugly wedged between the elevated tongue body and the maxillary central incisors. When this occurs, it is useful to **gently rotate the scope** slightly while moving the scope in the necessary direction.

In many cases, the desired view of the larynx will become visible only during the [i] productions as the tongue dorsum moves forward. However, some patients can tolerate the scope well enough that the laryngeal position during breathing may be observed. This is most likely if the **tongue anchoring** technique is employed.

c. **Tongue anchoring technique.** Frequently it is useful to anchor the tongue manually during performance of oral videoendoscopic examination of the larynx. This is performed by asking the patient to extend his or her tongue blade forward out of the mouth, wraping the tongue gently in a gauze cloth, and holding it firmly in place during the examination (Figure 5–5). This forward anchoring of the tongue assists patients who are otherwise unable to achieve a sufficiently anterior tongue position to permit observation of the entire length of the vocal folds. It

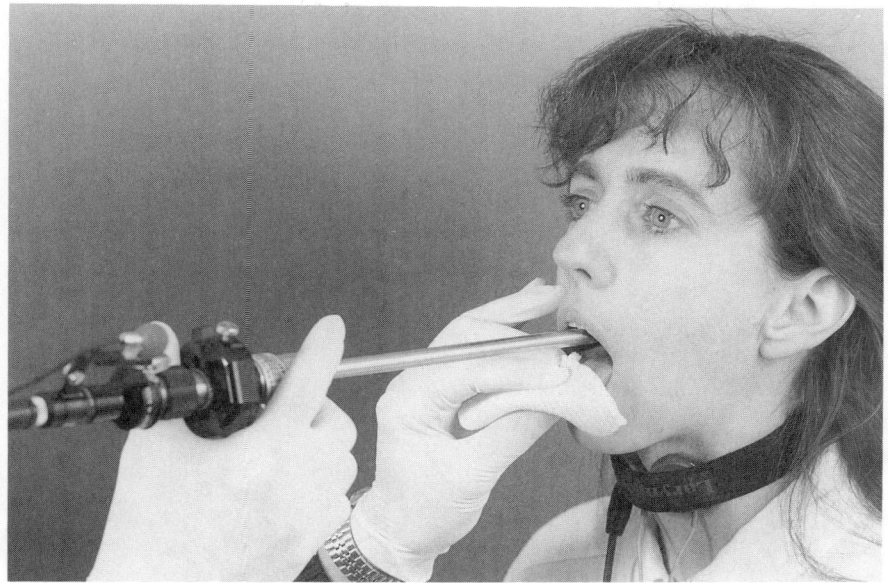

Figure 5–5. Use of the tongue anchor technique may improve visualization of the larynx by displacing the posterior tongue forward.

provides easier observation of vocal fold abduction for respiration if the clinician continues to anchor the tongue as the patient inspires between voice productions (Figure 5–6). If the tongue is released during respiration, it may move posteriorly and obscure the larynx from view.

2. Minimizing the Gag Reflex

As stated previously, some clinicians advocate the use of oral anesthetics to desensitize the patient to the oral scope and, therefore, minimize the gag reflex. This may be accomplished by spraying anesthesia into the patient's oral cavity as he or she maintains a mouth open posture. Deeper anesthesia may be accomplished by having the patient gargle an anesthesia solution. **The most important tools for minimizing gag,** however, are proper patient positioning and a good insertion technique by a steady clinical hand.

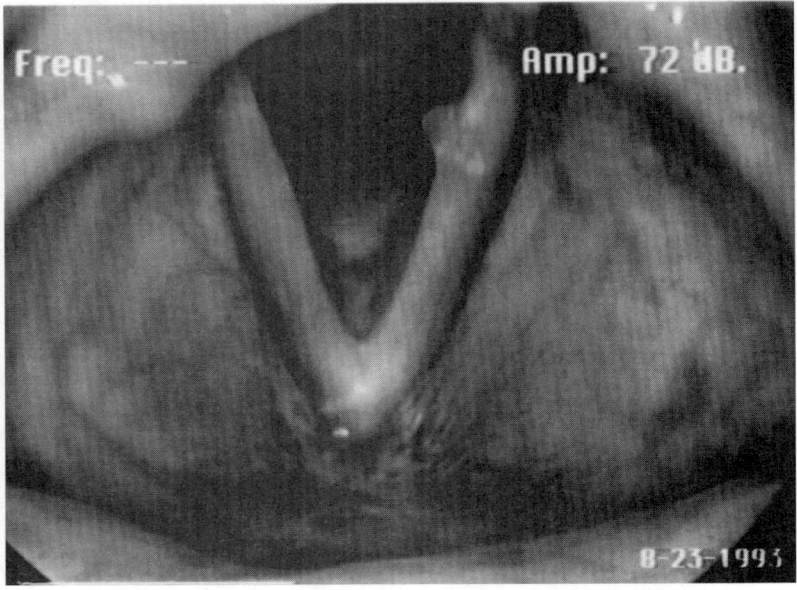

Figure 5–6. Visualization of the vocal folds in the fully abducted position during respiration is facilitated by continuing the tongue anchor technique after phonation has ended.

II. LARYNGEAL ASSESSMENT

Some of the practical observations in laryngeal videoendoscopic assessment were mentioned briefly in the description of procedures. Additional details will be provided here to describe what observations should be included.

Videoendoscopy and stroboscopic assessment of laryngeal function for voice **require a solid background in normal laryngeal anatomy and physiology**. That substantial area of study is beyond the scope of this volume. It will be assumed here that anyone interested in learning to do endoscopy will have acquired the requisite background.

Laryngeal assessment can be divided into nonstroboscopic and stroboscopic assessment. These refer to the different observations made when the stroboscopic light is and is not in use.

A. Nonstroboscopic Laryngeal Assessment

Nonstroboscopic laryngeal assessment begins when the endoscope is positioned to visualize the larynx. Because this part of the assessment is usually more extensive when performing **nasal videoendoscopy**, the discussion will focus on assessment when that technique is used.

Overall assessment of the structure and symmetry of the larynx may be assessed when the scope is positioned in the oropharynx just above the epiglottis. It is usually possible from that perspective to view the condition of the **major laryngeal structures, including the epiglottis, aryepiglottic folds, the ventricular folds, the arytenoids, and the true vocal folds.**

Arytenoid movement symmetry may be assessed by having the patient whistle or repeat [hi hi hi] sequences. If a **recurrent laryngeal nerve paralysis** exists, it will usually be clearly apparent during this maneuver (Figure 5–7).

Presence and extent of **supraglottic compression** may also be assessed from the oropharyngeal perspective during sustained [i] voicing. This will indicate any tendency for the patient to approximate the supraglottic structures during phonation, such as the ventricular or aryepiglottic folds. Anterior displacement of the arytenoids may be observed in some patients. Any supraglottic compression represents a hyperfunctional tendency by the patient and may be purely functional or may be secondary to some organic pathology that impairs ability to achieve normal glottal closure for voice production (Figure 5–8).

Close-up inspection of the laryngeal surface mucosa should be performed with the flexible endoscope only after the patient has been instructed to avoid speaking or swallowing. Assuming the patient is capable of complying with these instructions, the endoscope can be carefully moved into the laryngeal vestibule. The presence of **edema**, **erythema**, or less subtle changes in **laryngeal mucosa** may be visualized and inspected provided the patient is still and the clinician can avoid contacting any laryngeal surface tissue with the endoscope. The presence of **nodules, polyps**, or other **pathology** affecting the configuration of the vibrating edges of the vocal folds can be evaluated best from this

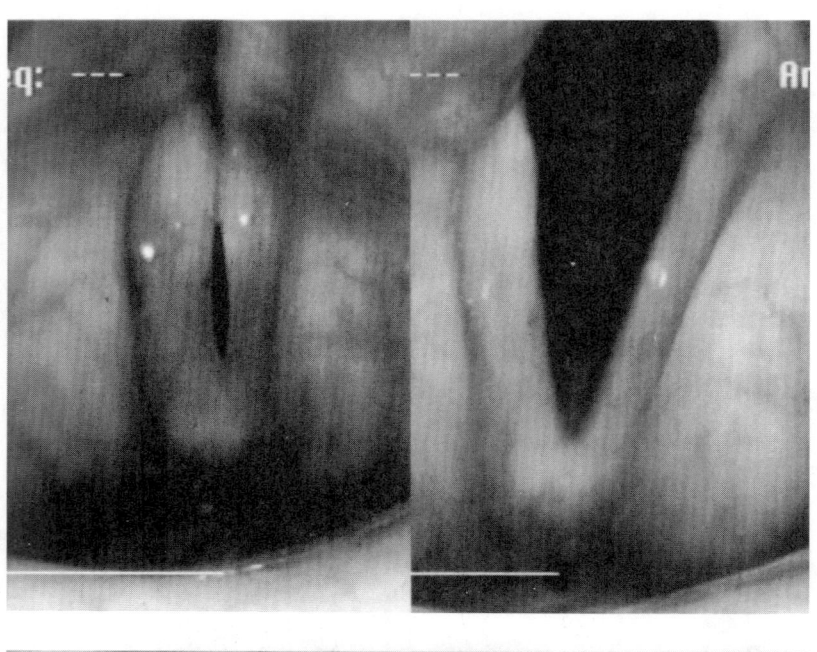

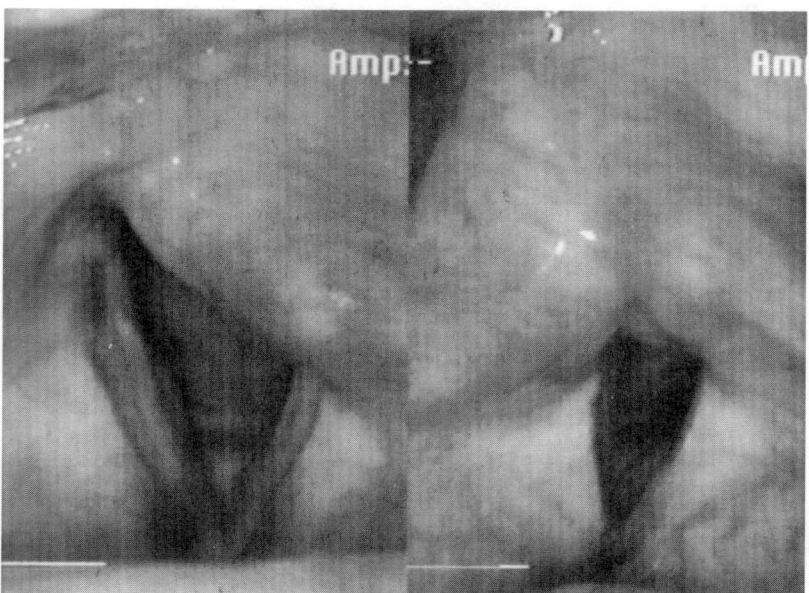

Figure 5–7. Recurrent laryngeal nerve paralysis is apparent on the right (**top**) in one patient and on the left (**bottom**) in another during successive adductor/abductor maneuvers.

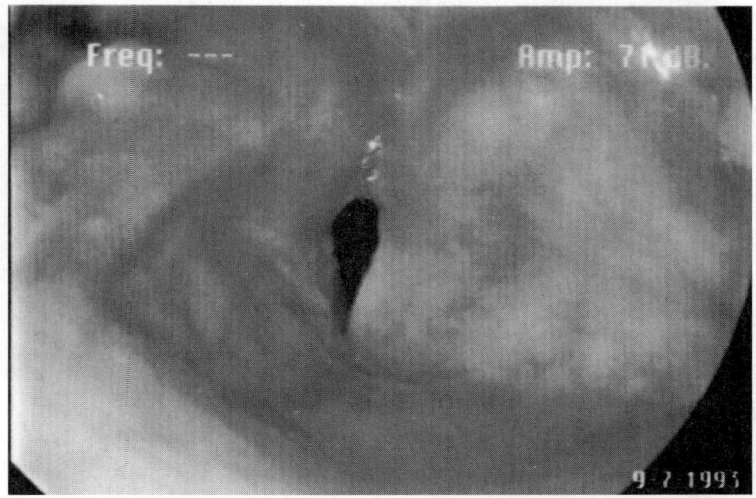

Figure 5–8. Severe supraglottic compression of the ventricular vocal folds during phonation may obscure the true vocal folds from view.

position (Figure 5–9). Some patients may be able to tolerate advancement of the scope to a level between the ventricular vocal folds. If so, the medial surfaces of the true vocal folds and the upper tracheal airway may be visualized. Any abnormalities in laryngeal surface structure, symmetry, and character should be noted and demonstrated on the videotape record.

B. Stroboscopic Laryngeal Assessment

Stroboscopy has matured as diagnostic tool for **assessment of vocal fold vibratory activity** (Hirano & Bless, 1993; Kitzing, 1985; Sataloff, Spiegel, & Hawkshaw, 1991). It has been found to be medically useful in the diagnosis, assessment, and treatment of many laryngeal pathologies including **cancer** (Wallesch, Sieron, & Johannsen, 1991; Zhao, 1992), **vocal fold paralysis** (Grundfast & Harley, 1989; Sercarz, Berke, Ming, & Gerratt, 1992; Slavit & Maragos, 1992; Watterson, McFarlane, & Menicucci, 1990), **trauma** (Ptok, 1993), **thyroid disease** (Sataloff, 1991), **spasmodic dysphonia** (Ford, Bless, & Lowery, 1990), **allergy,** (Dixon, 1992) and **central nervous system dysfunction** (Hacki et al., 1990). It is commonly used in the assessment of functional voice disorders and in evaluation of results of voice therapy (Kruse, 1989; Pluzhnikov, Lopatko, & Ibrakhem, 1992).

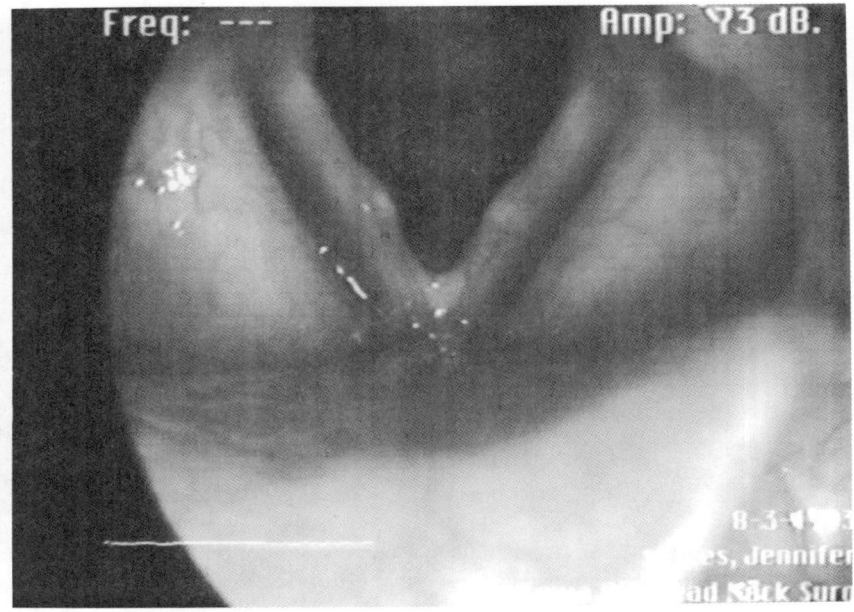

A

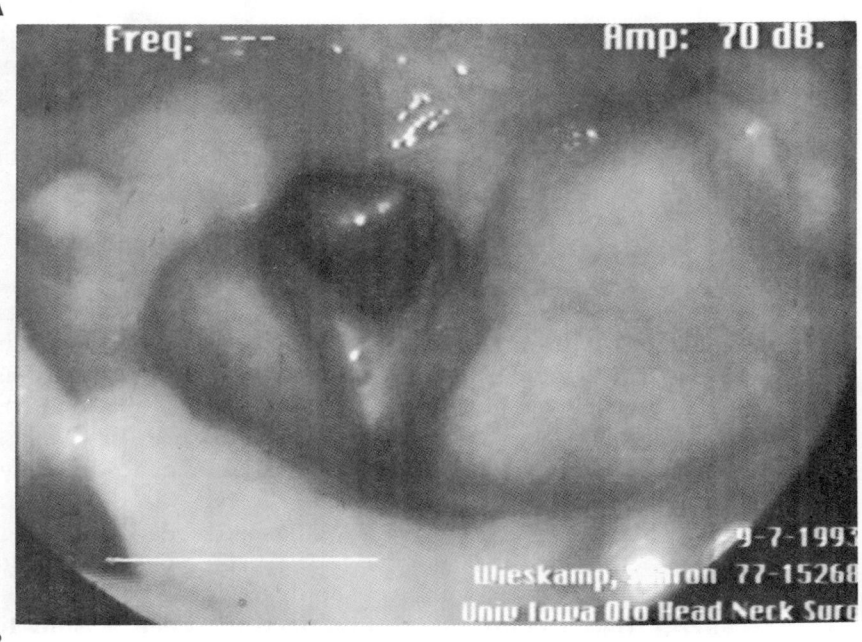

B

Figure 5–9. Inspection of the true vocal folds after instructing the patient not to speak or swallow may provide the best record of vocal fold tissue changes such

108

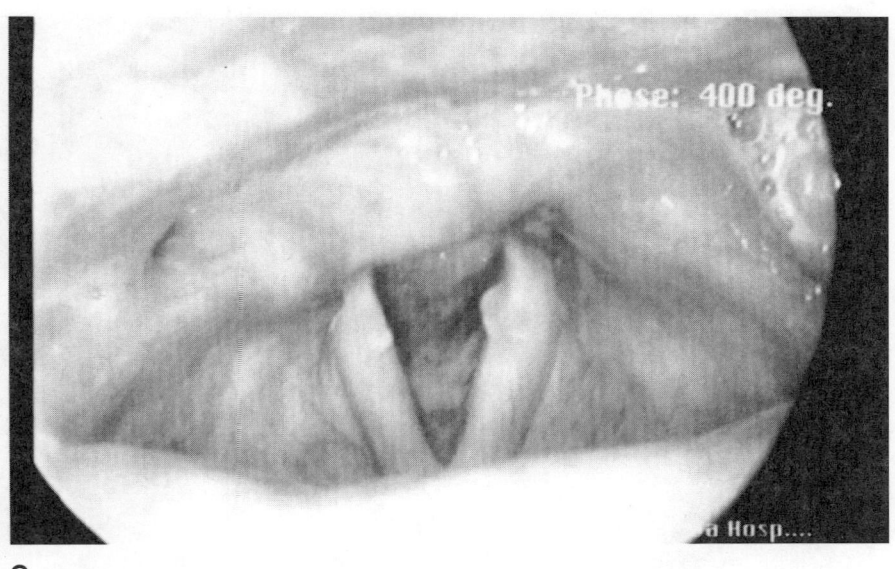

C

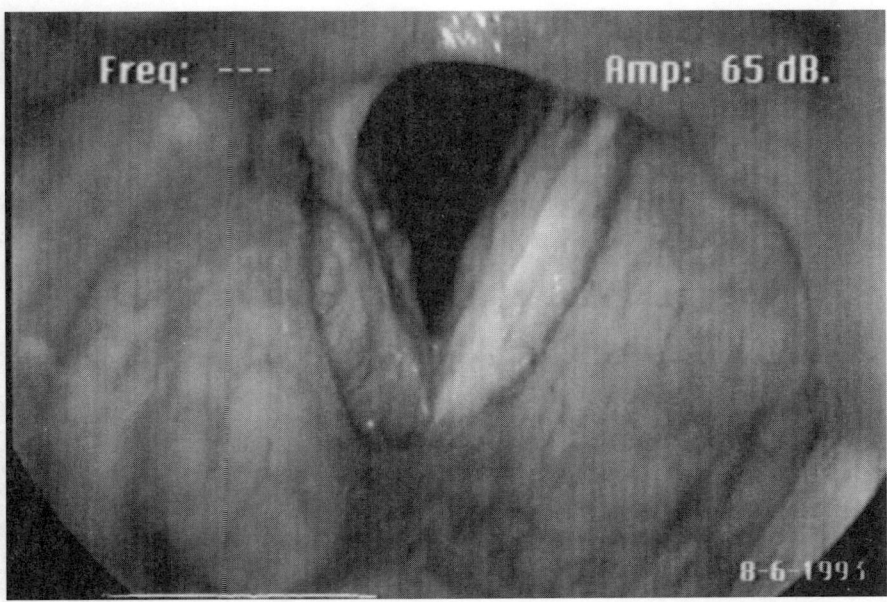

D

as bilateral nodules (**A**), anterior commisure webbing (**B**), left contact granuloma (**C**), right teflon granuloma (**D**), *(continued)*

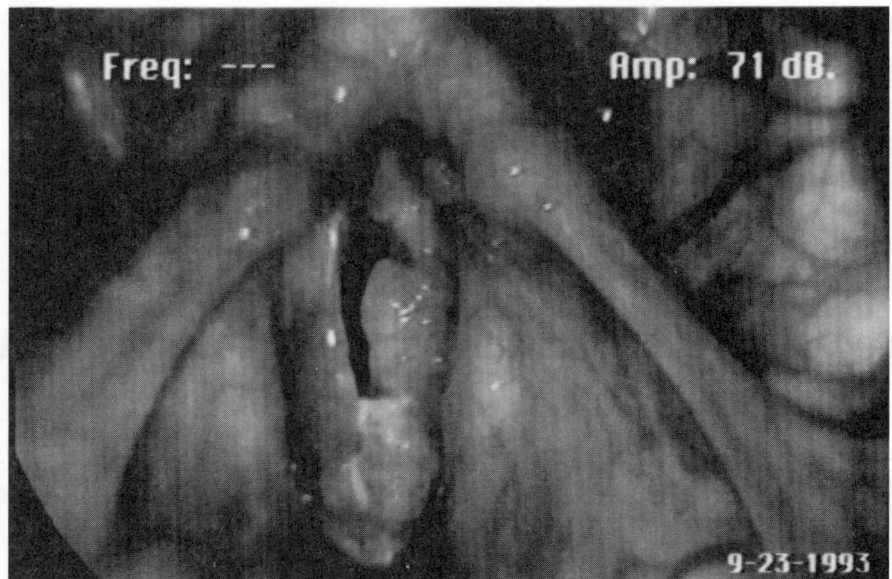

E

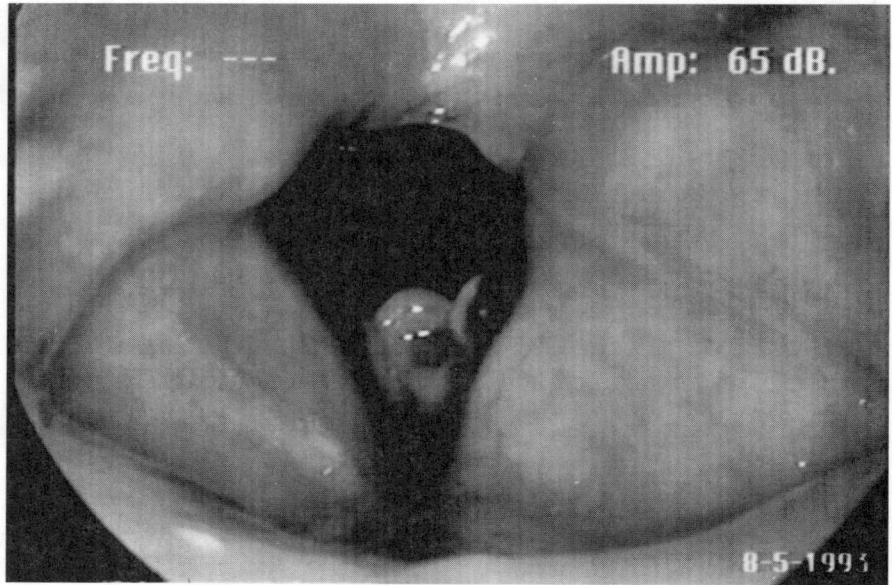

F

Figure 5–9. *(continued)* carcinoma (**E**), and hemorrhage post-traumatic thyroid fracture (**F**).

110

Stroboscopic assessment is usually **limited to the true vocal folds.** The standard observations include extent of glottal closure, relative amplitude of vocal fold vibration, symmetry of vibratory amplitude, phase symmetry, presence of nonvibrating segments, and presence and extent of the mucosal wave. Each of these observations is discussed below.

1. Extent of Glottal Closure

Extent of glottal closure may be assessed either during stroboscopic or nonstroboscopic assessment. Stroboscopic assessment is preferred because observations regarding extent of glottal closure should be pertinent to the **moment of maximum vocal fold contact**. During nonstroboscopic assessment, it is not possible to identify glottal configuration at any point during the vibratory cycle. Nonstroboscopic assessment of glottal closure is, therefore, less precise.

Glottal closure may be assessed in a number of ways. It may be described as either **complete, incomplete, or inconsistent.** More detail may be possible by rating or measuring the extent of residual glottal opening at the time of maximum closure as a proportion of maximum glottal opening (Karnell, Li, & Panje, 1991). Even more descriptive detail may be possible by identifying patterns of glottal closure, such as the **"hourglass" pattern**, as described originally by Bless (1987) and detailed more recently by Linville (1992). Examples of patients with varying degrees of glottal closure are shown in Figure 5–10. Examples of some of the measurements possible are demonstrated in Figure 5–11.

The approach to measurement demonstrated in Figure 5-11 employed **digital video processing**. The image of the vocal folds was computer digitized and measurements were made by manually tracing (using a "mouse") the glottal area, glottal length, and glottal width as shown in Figure 5–11A. In Figure 5–11B, measures taken at the moment of maximum glottal opening (image B–1) were used in the denominator of several ratio calculations that reflect the various aspects of glottal closure and vocal fold movement that occurred when the vocal folds moved toward the glottal midline (image B–2).

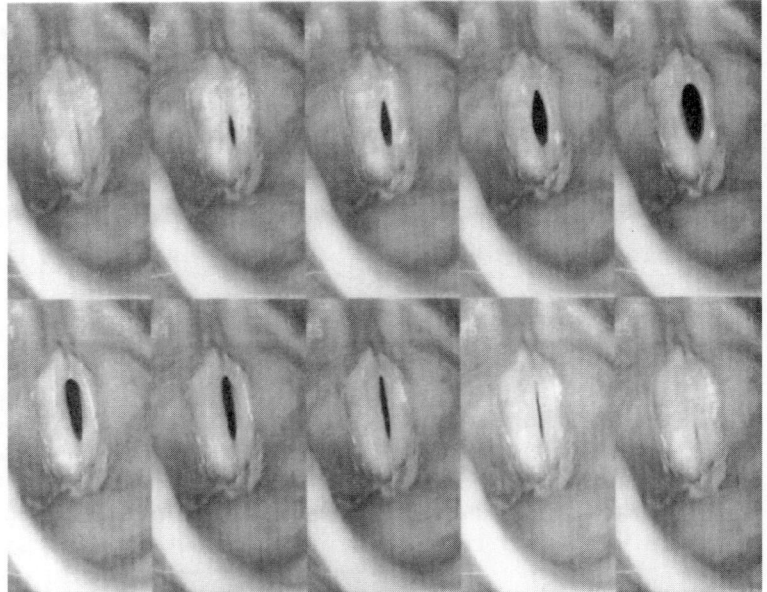

A

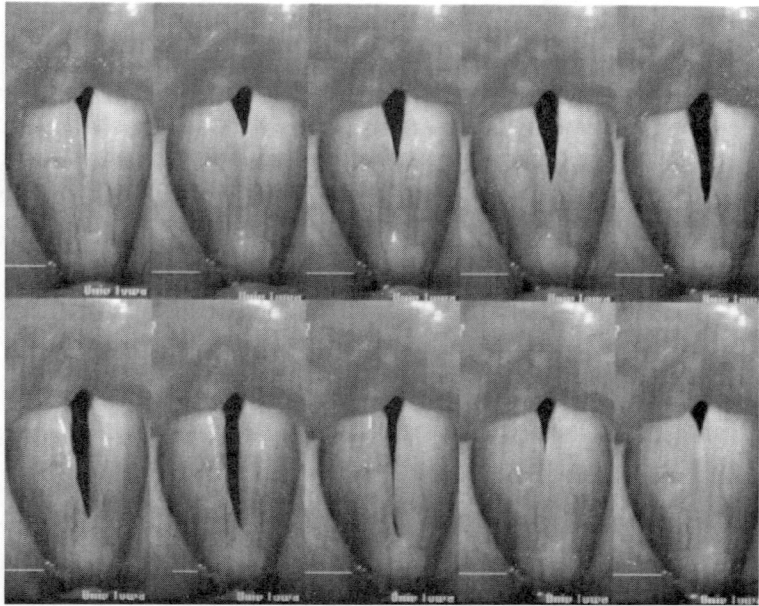

B

Figure 5–10. Varying degrees of maximum vocal fold closure may be observed during stroboscopic sequences including complete closure (upper left image in sequence **A**), and incomplete posterior closure (lower right in sequence **B**). The

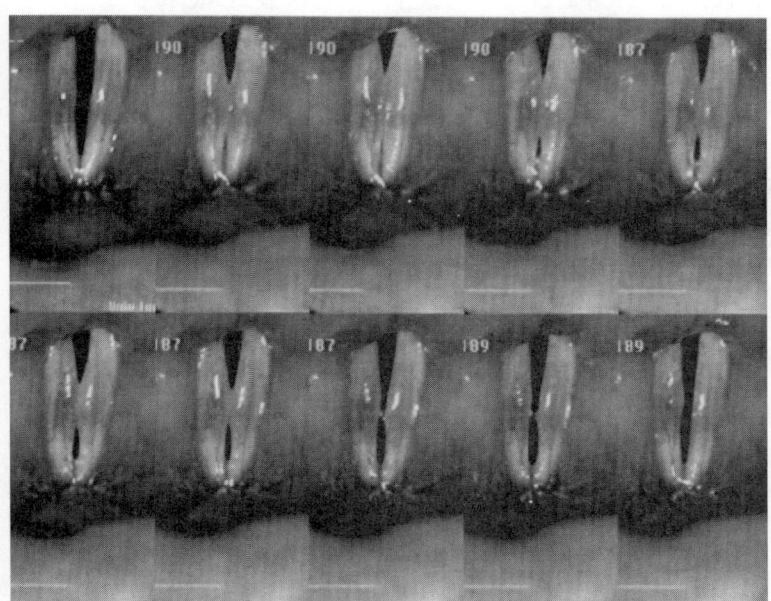

C

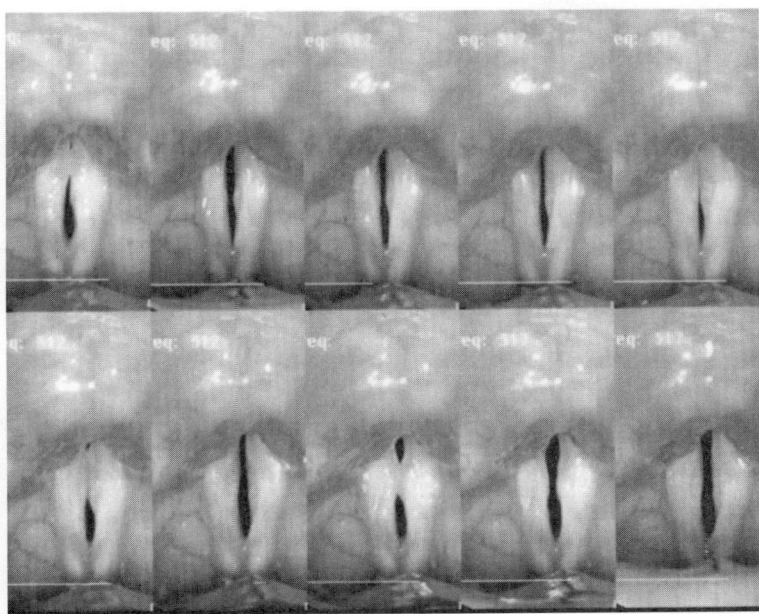

D

hourglass closure pattern is most commonly observed when vocal folds are between maximum opening and maximum closure (**C** and **D**).

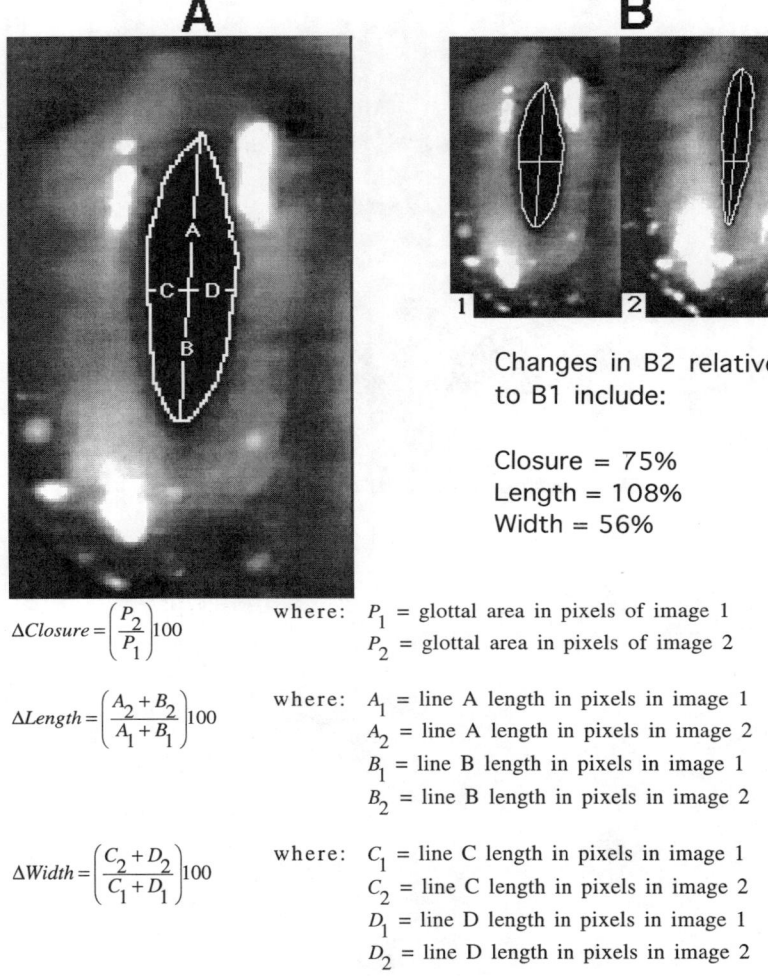

A

B

1 **2**

Changes in B2 relative
to B1 include:

Closure = 75%
Length = 108%
Width = 56%

$$\Delta Closure = \left(\frac{P_2}{P_1}\right)100$$

where: P_1 = glottal area in pixels of image 1
P_2 = glottal area in pixels of image 2

$$\Delta Length = \left(\frac{A_2 + B_2}{A_1 + B_1}\right)100$$

where: A_1 = line A length in pixels in image 1
A_2 = line A length in pixels in image 2
B_1 = line B length in pixels in image 1
B_2 = line B length in pixels in image 2

$$\Delta Width = \left(\frac{C_2 + D_2}{C_1 + D_1}\right)100$$

where: C_1 = line C length in pixels in image 1
C_2 = line C length in pixels in image 2
D_1 = line D length in pixels in image 1
D_2 = line D length in pixels in image 2

Figure 5–11. A relative measurement system for measuring glottal length, width, and opening.

2. Amplitude and Amplitude Symmetry of Vibration

Amplitude of vocal fold vibration refers to the extent of displacement of the medial edge of each vocal fold from midline observed at the time of maximum glottal opening. Similar to glottal closure, this may be rated using an equal appearing interval scale, measured relative to the glottal midline, or assigned to descriptive categories. An example of **amplitude asymmetry** is shown in Figure 5–12.

It is important to **assess both vocal folds' amplitude of vibration independently**. Differences in vocal fold tissue character between the two vocal folds may cause observable differences or asymmetries in amplitude of vibration. These differences may indicate the presence of subtle, yet significant, disease processes.

3. Phase Symmetry

Phase symmetry refers to the relative timing of motion of the vibrating vocal folds. If both folds reach the glottal midline at the same time and achieve maximum displacement away from the glottal midline at the same time, they are exhibit-

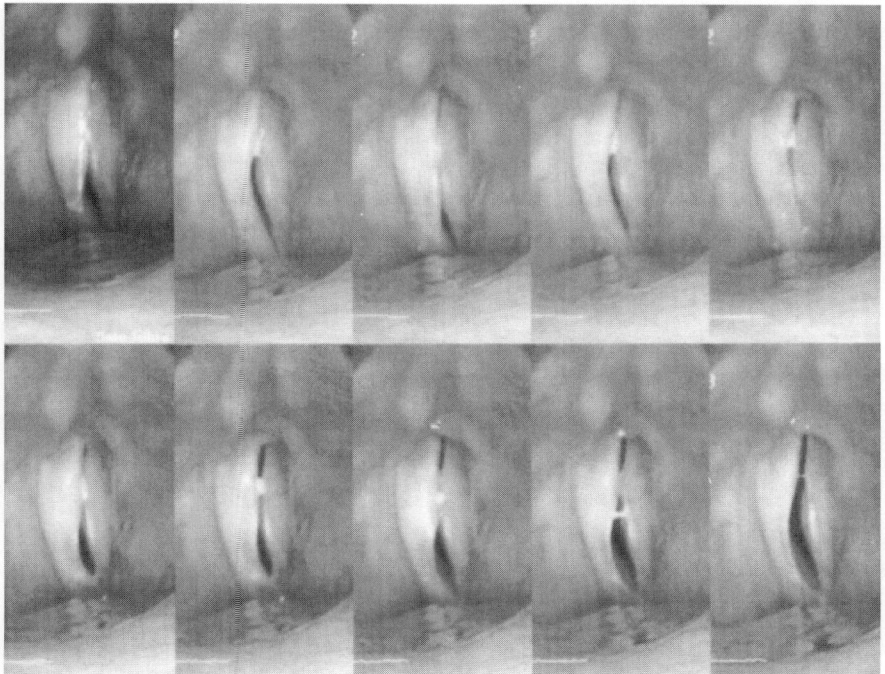

Figure 5–12. Vocal fold vibratory amplitude asymmetry. The right vocal fold moves laterally more than the left due to left vocal fold stiffness.

ing **normal phase symmetry**. However, if the vocal folds appear to reach these two vibratory extremes at different times, phase asymmetry exists (Figure 5–13). Like amplitude asymmetry, **phase asymmetry** reflects differences in tissue character between the vocal folds.

Phase symmetry is assessed most easily by judging whether the vibratory motions of the vocal folds appear **symmetrical, asymmetrical or inconsistently symmetrical**. More objective assessment requires field-by-field tracking of the position of the edges of the two vocal folds relative to the glottal midline (Von Leden et al., 1960).

4. Presence of Nonvibrating Segments

Vocal fold tissue should vibrate along the entire length of the membranous vocal fold during voice production. The presence of **tissue change** that affects all or part of a fold may

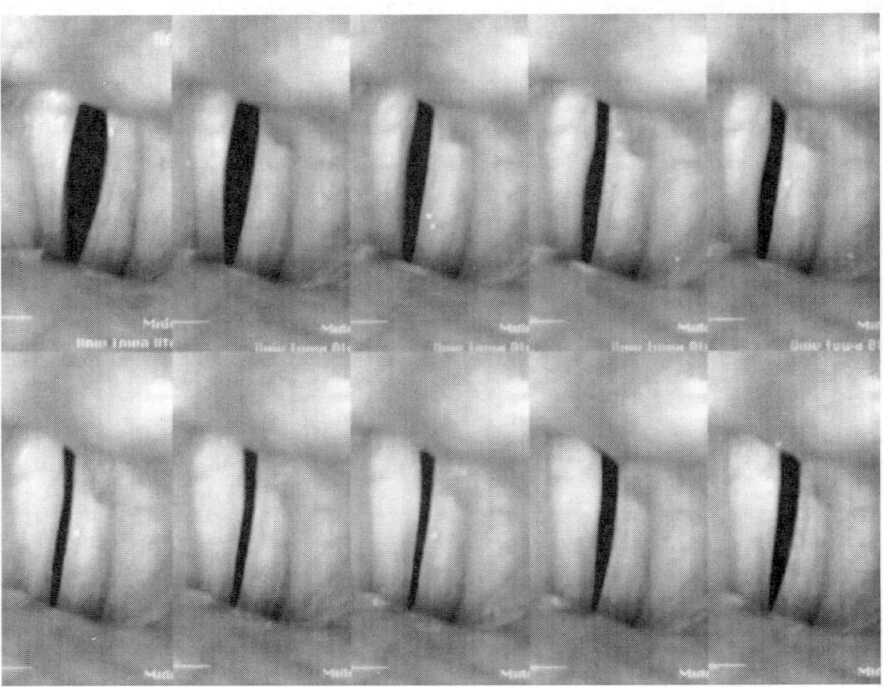

Figure 5–13. Vocal fold vibratory phase asymmetry in a patient with incomplete glottal closure.

result in failure of all or part of the vocal fold to move during phonation. Assessing the presence and the location of nonvibrating segments may provide clues regarding the nature of the underlying pathology and/or demonstrate the impact of a known pathology on vocal fold vibratory function.

5. Presence and Extent of the Mucosal Wave

The mucosal wave can be among the most difficult to assess phenomena of vocal fold vibration during videostroboscopy. The mucosal wave arises along the medial surface of the adducted vocal folds and, upon abduction, spreads laterally across the superior surface of the vocal folds. Accurate assessment requires excellent **laryngeal illumination** and adequate **video resolution**. For these reasons, it is frequently more difficult to assess when employing flexible fiberoptic endoscopy than when using rigid oral endoscopy.

A reduced or absent mucosal wave is frequently associated with increased stiffness of the vocal fold cover (Figure 5–14). **Variations in the mucosal wave may be among the first observable changes in vocal fold tissue** due to subtle, surface, tissue pathology. It may be assessed by applying rating scales or relative measurement schemes such as those employed for measuring vibratory amplitude. When these scales are applied to the mucosal wave, they refer to the distance from the medial edge of the vocal fold the mucosal wave appeared to travel during a typical vibratory cycle. Actual amplitude of the mucosal wave cannot be routinely assessed because it occurs along the sagittal axis which cannot be observed during endoscopic examination.

III. LIMITATIONS OF VIDEOSTROBOSCOPY

Video*endoscopic* examination of the larynx is useful for assessment and documentation purposes regardless of the severity of the associated voice disorder. The effectiveness of video*stroboscopy* is limited, however, by the **periodicity** of the patient's voice. If the patient's voice quality is severely dysphonic, there may not be sufficient periodicity in the voice signal to support adequate flashing of the stroboscopic light source. If the acoustic voice signal is highly aperiodic, so too will be the stroboscopic light flashing. When that occurs, the details of the vibratory movements of the vocal folds are obscured

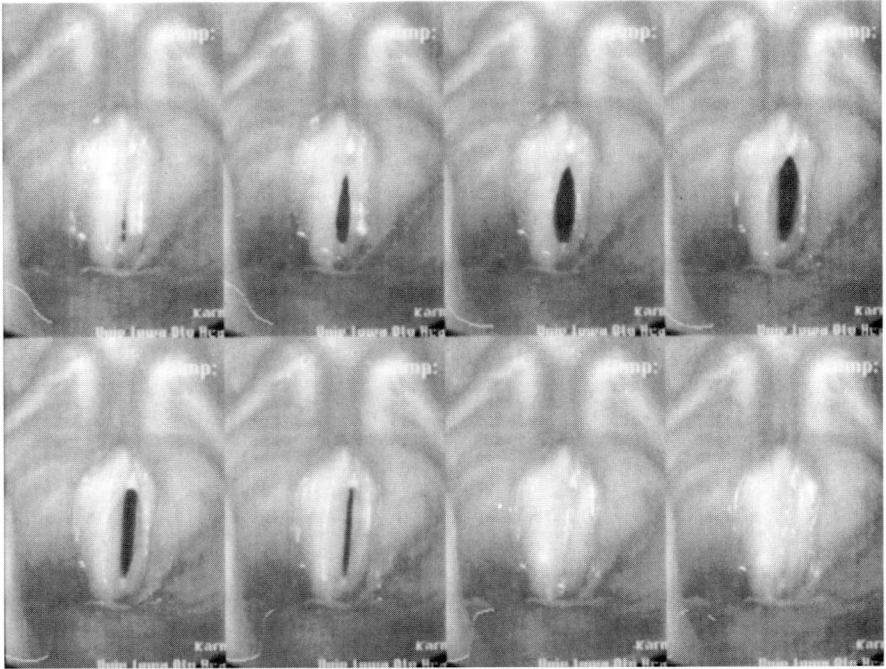

Figure 5–14. The mucosal wave appears clearly beginning in the upper right image along the patient's right vocal fold (the reader's left) and continuing in the first two images at the lower right as a line of reflected light which appears to move laterally away from the open glottis.

and limit what can be inferred about vibratory activity beyond the observation that it appears to be aperiodic. Videostroboscopy is most useful, therefore, in patients whose voice quality is mild-to-moderately impaired.

It should be stressed, however, that videostroboscopy is rarely important for the diagnostic/assessment process in patients with severely dysphonic voices. The physiologic correlates of more severe disorders are usually relatively obvious and visible during the nonstroboscopic videoendoscopic laryngeal examination. Videostroboscopy is most important in cases in which **pathology is subtle and not demonstrated adequately without observation of the vibratory pattern of the vocal folds.** These patients usually have mild-to-moderately dysphonic voices that are adequate for good quality videostroboscopic examination.

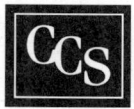

CHAPTER

6

Swallowing Videoendoscopy

E valuation and treatment of supraesophageal swallowing disorders has become a major responsibility of speech-language pathologists who work in medical settings. Videoendoscopy can be a useful tool for evaluating nonoral components of swallowing in select patients. This chapter will review the application of videoendoscopy for assessing swallowing.

I. PROCEDURES

Evaluation of selected aspects of swallowing is possible with nasally inserted, flexible endoscopy. A protocol for performing this evaluation has been advocated by Langmore and colleagues (1988). Referred to as "FEES" (*Fiberoptic Endoscopic Evaluation of Swallowing*) it has gained widespread acceptance. Elements of that protocol will be described here.

Although not intended to provide the same information as videofluorographic evaluation of swallowing (Langmore et al., 1988; Logemann, 1983), videoendoscopic swallowing assessment can provide

119

considerable information about the **structural condition of the pharynx and hypopharynx, the adequacy of the critical pharyngeal stage of swallowing, and the presence of aspiration.** The procedure has **several advantages over videofluoroscopy.** The equipment required for performing the procedure—flexible fiberoptic endoscope, light source, camera, and video tape recorder—can be moved to the patient's bedside if the patient is not ambulatory. The procedure is nonradiographic so that duration of the procedure may be determined by the complexity of the disorder and patient comfort rather than concerns about radiation exposure.

A. Anesthesia

Procedures for applying anesthesia in assessment of swallowing disorders are **identical to those for nasal videoendoscopy** for velopharyngeal or laryngeal assessment. A small amount of topical anesthetic and, if needed, vasoconstrictor may be applied to reduce patient discomfort. Also, application of lubricant to the side of the scope is useful to facilitate nasal insertion. No anesthesia should be applied to the oral cavity or pharynx. Desensitization of these areas may affect swallowing leading to spurious results.

B. Nasal Insertion

Insertion of the scope through the nasal passages may be performed as described for velopharyngeal and laryngeal evaluations. As with those applications, **middle nasal meatus insertion is preferable** when possible. This positioning allows for a higher perspective in the nasopharynx when observing the velopharyngeal mechanism during swallowing. It also encourages the flexible endoscope insertion tube to extend along the posterior pharyngeal wall when advanced into the oropharynx. Insertion through the inferior nasal meatus may result in unwanted scope movements during swallowing gestures due to velar elevation, because the scope is usually positioned upon the nasal surface of the soft palate.

C. Scope Positioning

There are three locations where the scope must be positioned at various times during a videoendoscopic swallowing examination (Figure 6–1A–C). The first position is in the **nasopharynx** and is intended to permit observation of velopharyngeal closure during swallowing gestures. This position is identical to that desired when velopharyngeal closure for speech production is being assessed. The second position is in the **oropharynx** above the level of the superior tip of the epiglottis and is intended to allow visualization of the pharynx before, during, and after the swallow maneuver. This position is identical to that desired when the goal is assessment of gross adductor/abductor motility of the larynx for voice production. The third position is within the **laryngeal vestibule** just superior to the ventricular folds and is intended to permit close inspection of the laryngeal vestibule for evidence of aspiration after a swallow has been completed. This position is identical to that desired when performing close inspection of the vocal fold tissue during a videoendoscopic voice evaluation.

II. SWALLOWING ASSESSMENT

The scope is positioned first in the nasopharynx for viewing the velopharyngeal mechanism. The patient is instructed to perform a "dry" (no water intake, saliva only) swallow while the clinician observes the velopharyngeal mechanism. Saliva may be colored by placing one or two drops of blue food color on the patient's tongue. **Complete velopharyngeal closure is expected during a normal swallow.** If closure is **incomplete**, as may be the case if a paralysis exists or if tissue loss due to pharyngeal cancer resection has occurred, **saliva** may be observed moving from the oral cavity through the velopharyngeal port into the **nasal cavity** during the swallow reflex. It is useful to observe the velopharyngeal port at this stage, particularly if the patient has reported symptoms of nasal reflux when swallowing. It is not advisable to give the patient a liquid bolus during the initial velopharyngeal evaluation. Introduction of a liquid bolus could result in aspiration that cannot be evaluated while the scope is positioned above the velopharyngeal port.

The endoscope is then advanced through the open velopharyngeal port while asking the patient to breath through the nasal cavity. Then, the patient may be instructed to sip and hold orally a small amount of ice chips or liquid colored with blue or green food coloring. The patient's posterior liqual-palatal seal may be inadequate if **material is observed prematurely falling into the pharynx** during this oral hold maneuver.

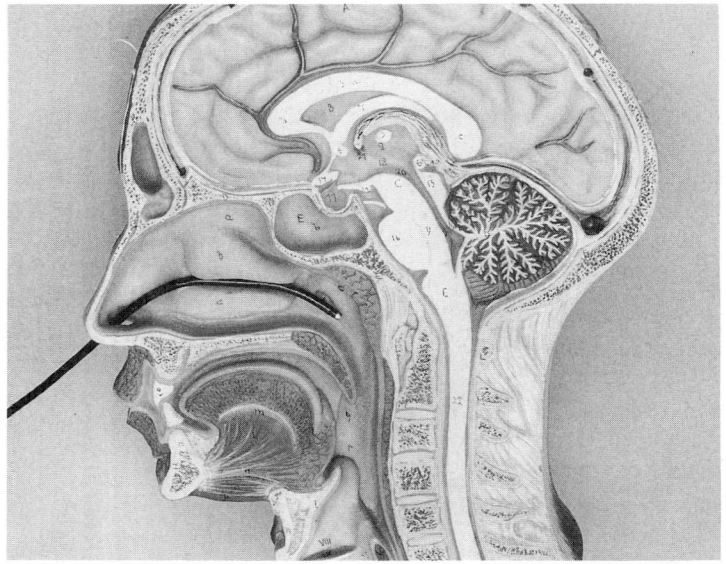

A

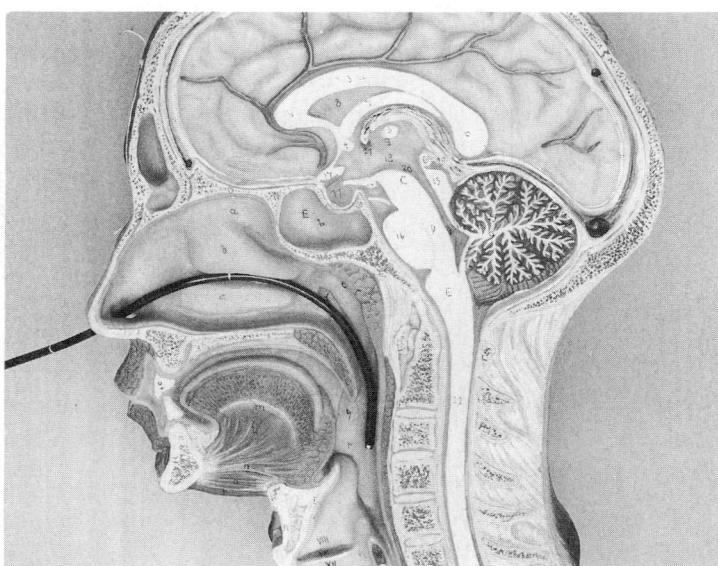

B

Figure 6–1. Flexible nasal endoscopic examination of swallowing is performed during the swallow while the scope is positioned in the nasopharynx (**A**) and oropharynx (**B**). The scope may be advanced into the largyngeal vestibule

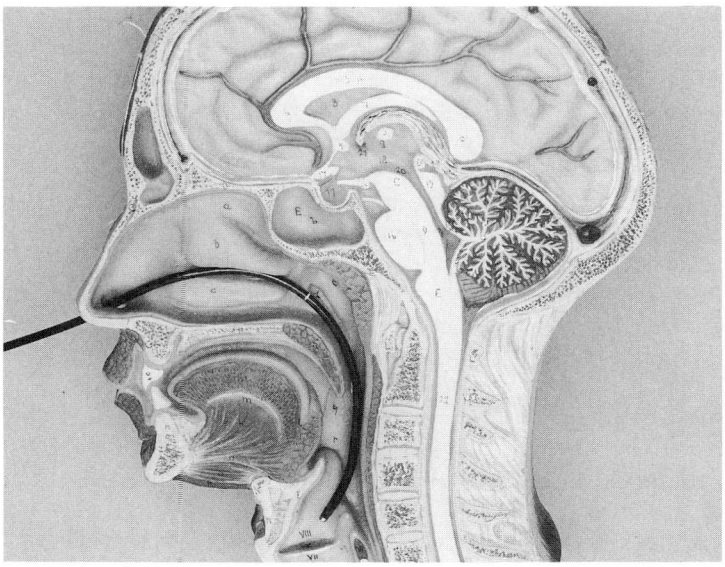

C

(**C**) during respiration for close inspection before or after the swallow.

Next, the patient should be instructed to swallow. A normal swallow appears as a very rapid sequence of events, including **laryngeal elevation, posterior displacement of the epiglottis, and velopharyngeal elevation** which, together, serve to obscure the endoscopic view momentarily. However, if the swallow reflex is weak, the epiglottis may not invert and the view of the pharynx may be maintained during the reflex.

Evaluation after the swallow involves **close inspection of the hypopharynx** for residual liquid pooling in the pyriform sinuses and valleculae after the swallow. This material should be watched closely due to the risk of spillage into the laryngeal vestibule after the swallow. **Close inspection of the laryngeal vestibule** should follow as soon as the patient is breathing comfortably after the swallow. The colored liquid may temporarily stain the pharyngeal surface of the epiglottis, the superior surface of the ventricular folds, and the superior surface of the true vocal folds if vestibular or tracheal aspiration occurred. **Tracheal aspiration** can frequently be confirmed by examining the walls of the trachea just below the true vocal folds for staining. The tracheal walls can usually be observed while the flexible scope is positioned in the laryngeal vestibule just above the ventricular folds. The clinician must be careful to **caution the patient not to speak or swallow during close inspection**, however, in order to avoid stimulating a cough or gag reflex.

Additional swallows of stained materials of varying consistencies (paste, cookie, etc.) also may be evaluated in a similar manner after the scope is removed to the level of the oropharynx. Close inspection of the hypopharynx and laryngeal trachea is necessary between each swallow. As with any evaluation of swallowing, **evidence of gross aspiration is indication for terminating the study**.

Experimentation with compensatory maneuvers such as **head turn, chin tuck, supraglottic swallow**, or **Mendelsohn maneuver** may be attempted to assess the usefulness of these techniques for controlling aspiration. It is advisable to train the patient to perform these maneuvers prior to insertion of the endoscope so that simple verbal instructions will be more likely to generate the appropriate behavior once the scope is in place. The clinician must be careful to move the position of the scope as the patient's head moves in order to maintain the desired position of the scope in the pharynx and avoid patient discomfort.

Evaluation of hypopharyngeal and laryngeal sensitivity to tactile stimulation may be indicated in patients who appear to be insensitive to aspiration or pyriform sinus residue. This is possible by advancing the endoscope and lightly touching the ventricular folds and/or the true vocal folds with the tip of the scope. Normal reaction should be a reflexive gag or cough; thus the clinician should be prepared to remove the endoscope from the laryngeal vestibule quickly and possibly from the patient altogether if the reaction results in severe head and shoulder movements. Obviously, this part of the evaluation **should always be the last component** of the endoscopic swallowing evaluation. Scope contact with the surfaces of the laryngeal vestibule should be avoided in patients who appear to be sensitive to aspiration and in patients who do not demonstrate evidence of aspiration.

The results of the endoscopic swallowing evaluation may be sufficient to warrant recommendation of dietary modification, therapeutic techniques, or both. This is particularly true if the patient is unable to be moved or cannot otherwise tolerate a more detailed swallowing evaluation. Evidence of abnormal swallowing observed during an endoscopic examination is considered grounds for referral for a **videofluorographic oropharyngeal motility study** (OPM, a.k.a. modified barium swallow or cookie swallow) whenever possible.

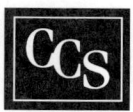

CHAPTER

7

Supplementary Techniques

V ideoendoscopic imaging of the speech production mechanism is a power-
ful clinical tool. However, there are some inherent limitations which can
be minimized to some extent by using supplementary techniques. Two such
techniques, endoscopy with photodetection and videostroboscopy with synchronized electroglottography, will be described briefly.

I. VELOPHARYNGEAL VIDEOENDOSCOPY WITH
PHOTODETECTION

Videoendoscopic evaluation of velopharyngeal closure is usually
successful in identifying the extent and timing of inappropriate velopharyngeal opening during speech production. However, given the
two-dimensional nature of its images, there are times when uncertain-
ties exist. In such cases, the use of photodetection with endoscopy may
be useful.

Photodetection as a technique for evaluation of velopharyngeal valving
during speech has been described in the literature (Dalston, 1982,

1989; Dalston & Seaver, 1990; Keefe & Dalston, 1989; Kunzel, 1982). It employs two small, fiberoptic fibers inserted nasally. One fiber, attached to an external light source, is inserted through the **velopharyngeal port into the oropharynx**. The other, attached to an external photodiode, is positioned **above the velopharyngeal area in the nasopharynx**. This configuration allows the light transmitted through the velopharyngeal port from the orally positioned light-emitting fiber to be picked up by the nasally positioned fiber attached to the photodiode. By observing the output of the photodiode on an oscilloscope, variations in velopharyngeal valving may be observed.

An **integrated endoscopy/photodetection system** (Karnell & Seaver, 1993) uses a variation of the photodetection approach. This system employs a pediatric bronchoscope (Olympus BF-3C20) with a 3.7 mm outside diameter (o.d.) insertion tube to obtain endoscopic images of the velopharyngeal structures. Within the endoscope insertion tube is a 1.2 mm inside diameter (i.d.) instrument channel through which a single fiberoptic fiber is inserted. The overall outside diameter of the endoscope is 3.7 mm.

An RCA photodiode is coupled to the fiberoptic fiber. This fiber serves as the photodetector component of the system. A 1 cm length at the distal end of the light detecting fiber is gently abraded to remove the outer fiber coating and, therefore, increase light pickup sensitivity. Also, the distal end of the fiber is modified to create a small, reflective bulb.

With the endoscope positioned in the **nasopharynx**, the photodetection fiber is extended through the velopharyngeal port into the **oropharynx**. Light from the endoscope strikes the bulb on the tip of the photodetection fiber and is reflected, in part, back to the light sensitive 1 cm abraded segment of the fiber. The endoscope-light fiber portion of the system is shown in Figure 7–1.

The photodiode output voltage signal is low-pass filtered at 40 Hz, amplified 20 dB (Wavetek model 432 Hi-Lo filter with internal amplifier), and displayed on a laboratory oscilloscope (Tektronix model 2220). The polarity of the oscilloscope display may be reversed so that the direction of the beam movement corresponds with velopharyngeal structural movements (i.e., upward beam deflection represented less light detection by the photodiode and less oscilloscopic voltage due to more velopharyngeal closure). The oscilloscopic display may be recorded along with the endoscopic image using a split-screen

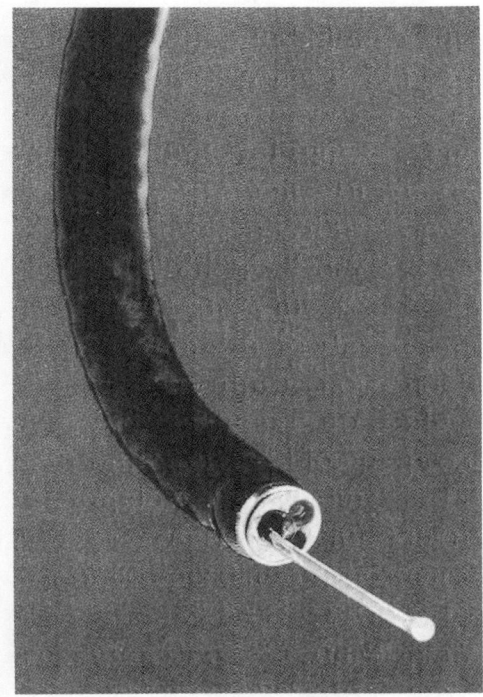

Figure 7–1. The distal tip of the insertion tube of an endoscope (Olympus BF-3C20) with internal instrument channel through which a photodetector light fiber is inserted.

videotape recording system (Panasonic model AG-7300 video recorder, Sony KX 1211 HG video monitor, Sony AVC-3260 camera, Meade Electronic Custom Video Clock, Sony SEG 1-A special effects generator).

Examples of variations in photodetector output during "Come to my house tonight for ice cream cake" are shown in Figure 7–2A–B. A three-level scale is included in each image showing beam position during maximum light (lowest line on scale), minimum light (light out condition, top line of scale), and 50% between the maximum and minimum is shown next to the photodetector beam. The beam position associated with each endoscopic image is shown next to the scale in each image. The subject with normal speech shown in 7–2A achieved complete closure during each maximum closure gesture. However, the subject with mild hypernasality shown in 7–2B failed to achieve closure consistently during the maximum closure gestures.

Currently, integrated videoendoscopy and photodetection is an **experimental technique**. Initial reports have shown, however, that it has

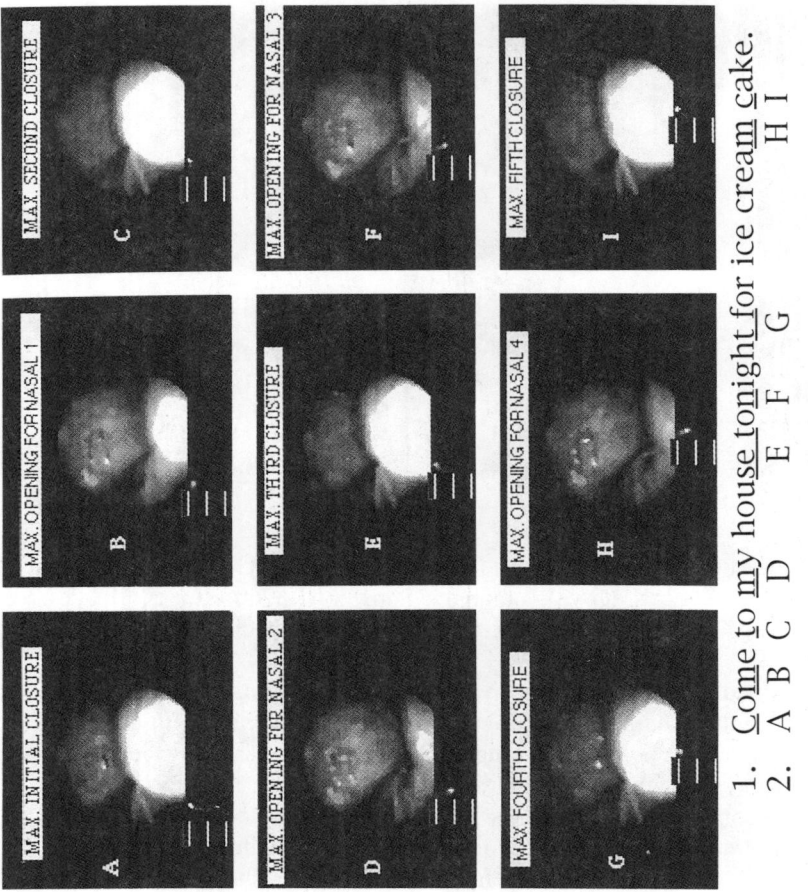

MAX. INITIAL CLOSURE   A

MAX. OPENING FOR NASAL 1   B

MAX. SECOND CLOSURE   C

MAX. OPENING FOR NASAL 2   D

MAX. THIRD CLOSURE   E

MAX. OPENING FOR NASAL 3   F

MAX. FOURTH CLOSURE   G

MAX. OPENING FOR NASAL 4   H

MAX. FIFTH CLOSURE   I

1. Come to my house tonight for ice cream cake.

2. A B C D   E F G   H I

A

130

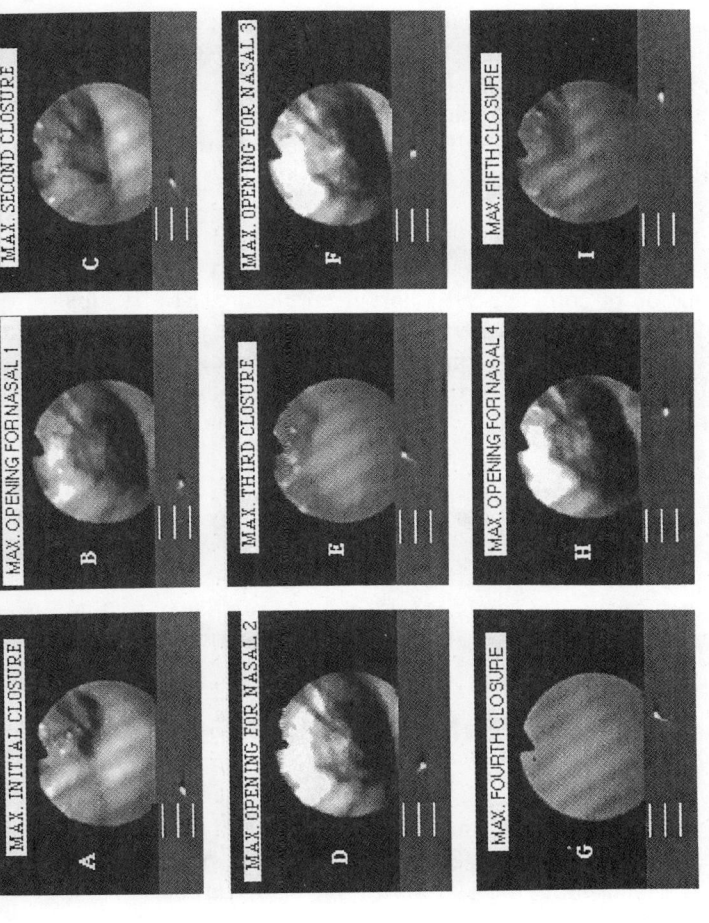

1. Come to my house tonight for ice cream cake.
2. A B C D   E F G   H I

B

Figure 7–2. Examples of the split screen video display are shown in a subject with normal speech (**A**) and a subject with mild hypernasality (**B**).

promise as a clinical tool for evaluating velopharyngeal closure. For example, Karnell, Seaver, and Dalston (1988) reported that the photodetector output is consistent with videoendoscopic observations of velopharyngeal opening and closing gestures during transitions from oral to nasal speech sound segments. Covello, Karnell, and Seaver (1992) reported that the photodetector output was linear but that specific controls regarding the relative position of the fiber and the endoscope must be in place to assure optimal system performance. Most importantly, the system has been shown to be **sensitive to momentary, abnormal breaches in velopharyngeal closure** that may occur in the speech of patients with inconsistent or marginal velopharyngeal insufficiency (Karnell & Seaver, 1993; Karnell, Seaver, & Dalston, 1988).

Most recently, Karnell and Seaver (1993) demonstrated how a **"light out"** condition may be used to establish a criterion level for photodetector confirmation of complete velopharyngeal closure. Briefly, this involves recording of the photodetector output when the system is in place and the endoscopic light is momentarily turned off. Theoretically, the photodetector output during the light off condition should be similar to photodetector output when complete velopharyngeal closure is achieved.

Additional clinical testing of integrated videoendoscopy and photodetection will be necessary before the system becomes useful for routine clinical applications. In particular, smaller diameter flexible endoscopes with insertion channels must be made available so that patients with very small nasal lumens may be evaluated.

II. VIDEOSTROBOSCOPY WITH SYNCHRONIZED ELECTROGLOTTOGRAPHY

Synchronized videostroboscopy and electroglottography is gaining widespread acceptance as a clinical evaluation tool. This system, originally described by Anastaplo and Karnell (1988) and Karnell (1989), provides a means for determining how **electroglottographic signals and videostroboscopic images relate to each other**.

The original system included a Bruel and Kjaer Model 4914 stroboscopic light source which performed two functions simultaneously. First, it enabled recording of videostroboscopic images of vocal fold movements during phonation. The stroboscopic light source also served to trigger a Tektronix Type 502-1 dual screen oscilloscope used to display an EGG signal from a Synchrovoice Research Electroglottograph. No filtering of the electroglottographic waveform was used to avoid phase distortion between the videostroboscopic images and the EGG waveform. More recently, EGG equipment incorporating zero phase filtering and amplification is available (Glottal Enterprises) and can provide a more stable EGG waveform.

A video image of the EGG oscilloscope screen was produced by focusing an Ikegami Model ITCC-46 video camera on the oscilloscope display. The video outputs from this camera and the videostroboscopic camera were displayed simultaneously on a Sony Model KX-1211 HG video monitor via an RCA video splitter. The result was a split screen image showing the stroboscopic image at the middle of the monitor screen and the triggered EGG image near top or the bottom of the screen (Figure 7–3).

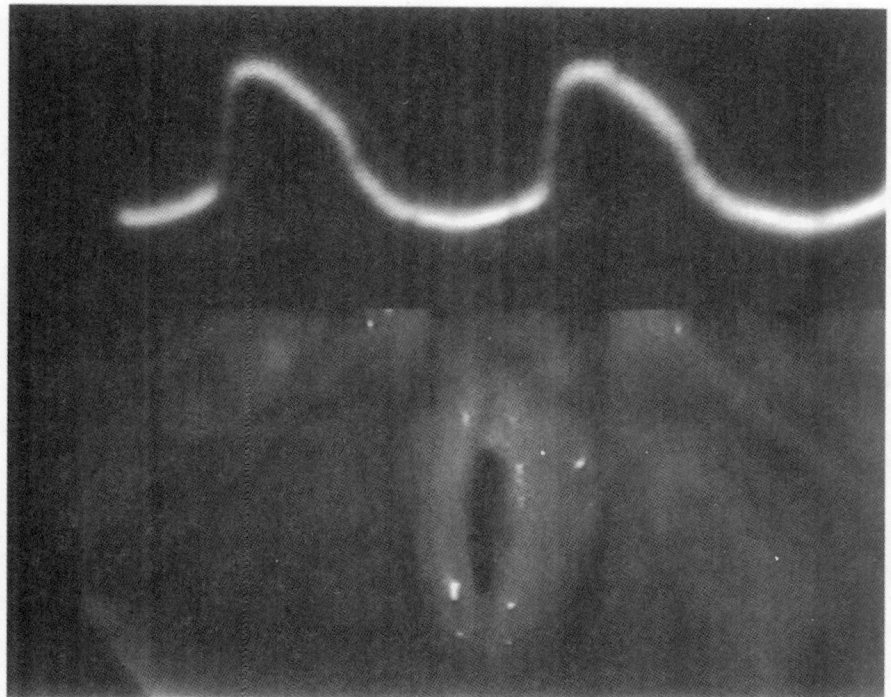

Figure 7–3. Split screen synchronized videostroboscopic image of the vocal folds and the electroglottographic waveform.

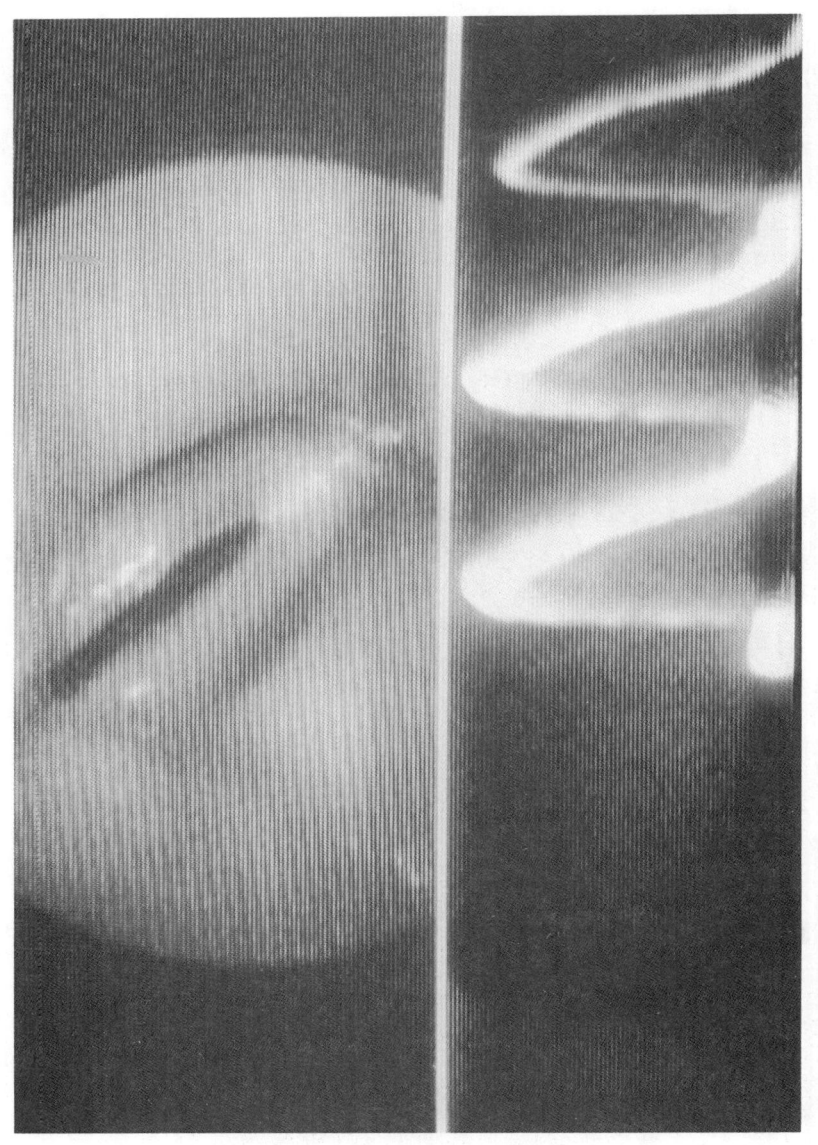

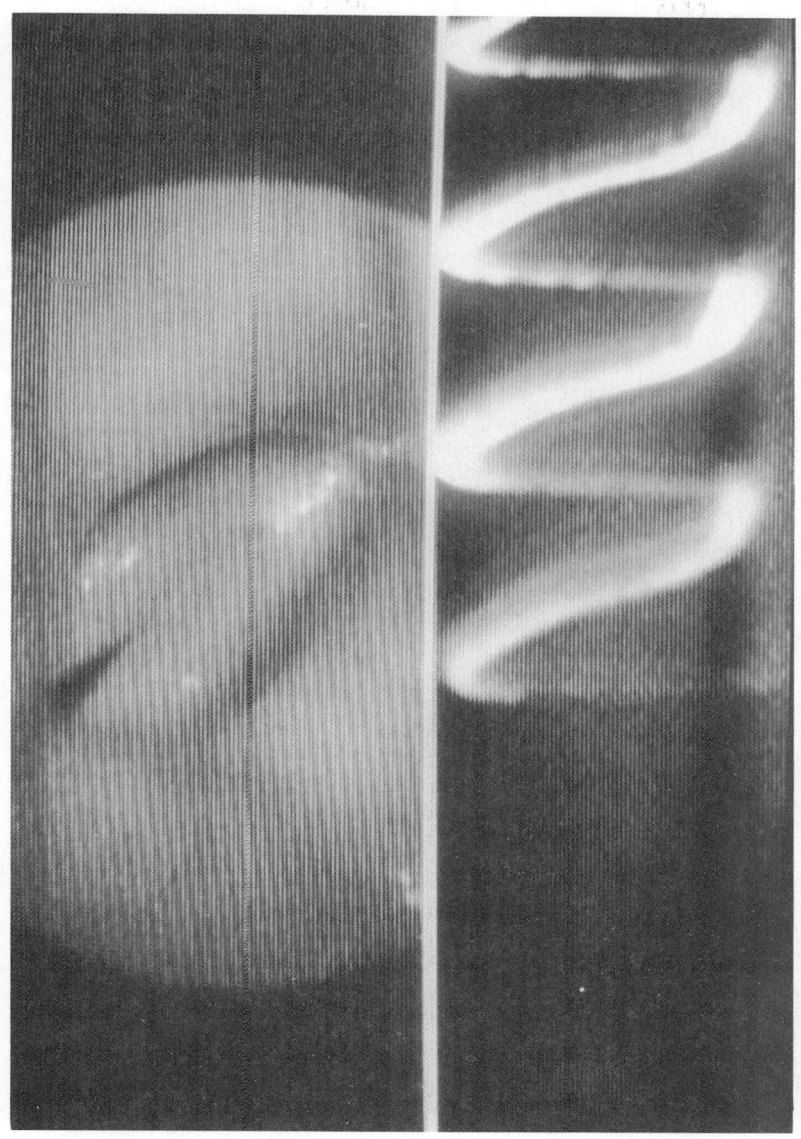

Figure 7–4. A sequence of synchronized videostroboscopic/electroglottographic images during a phonatory cycle. The left-most edge of the waveform corresponds to the glottal configuation (*continued*)

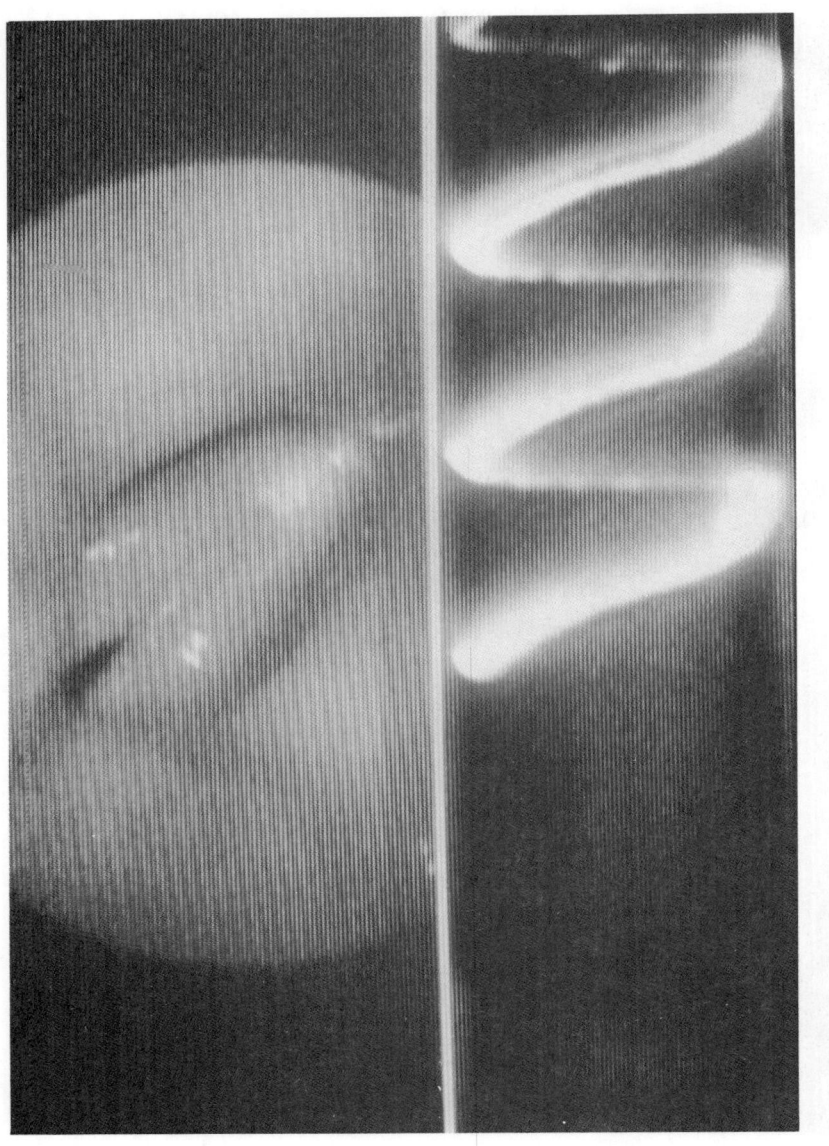

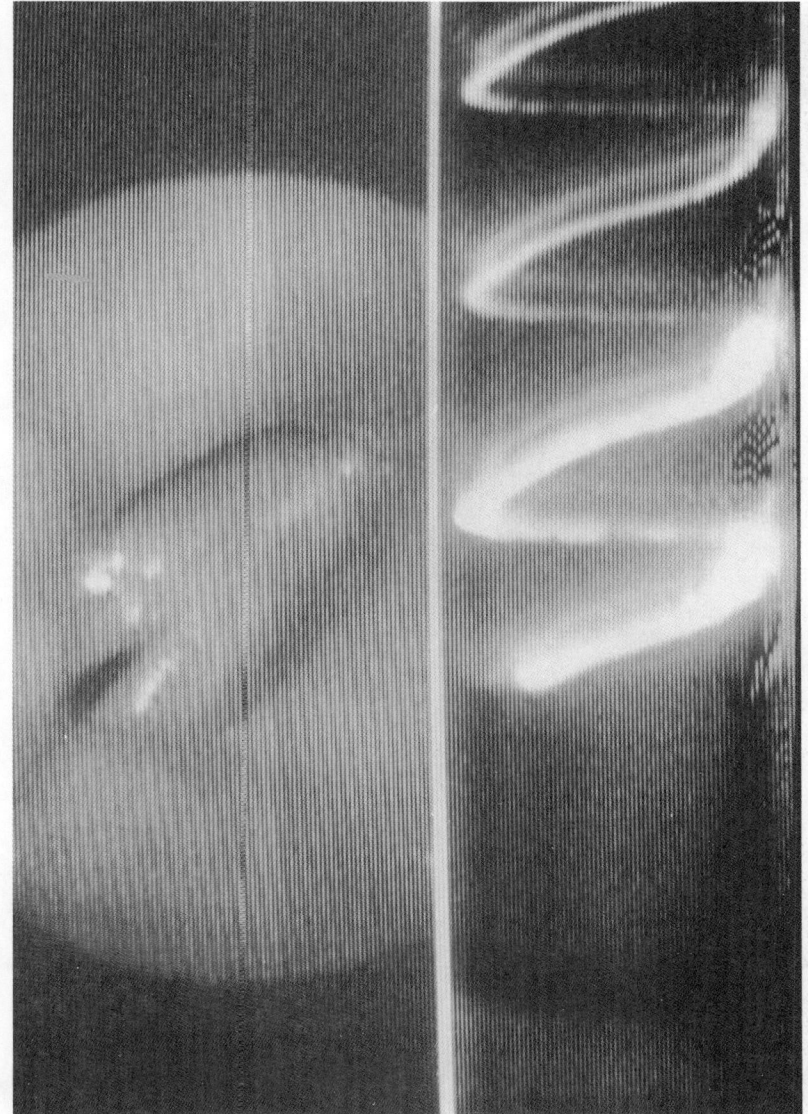

Figure 7-4. (continued)

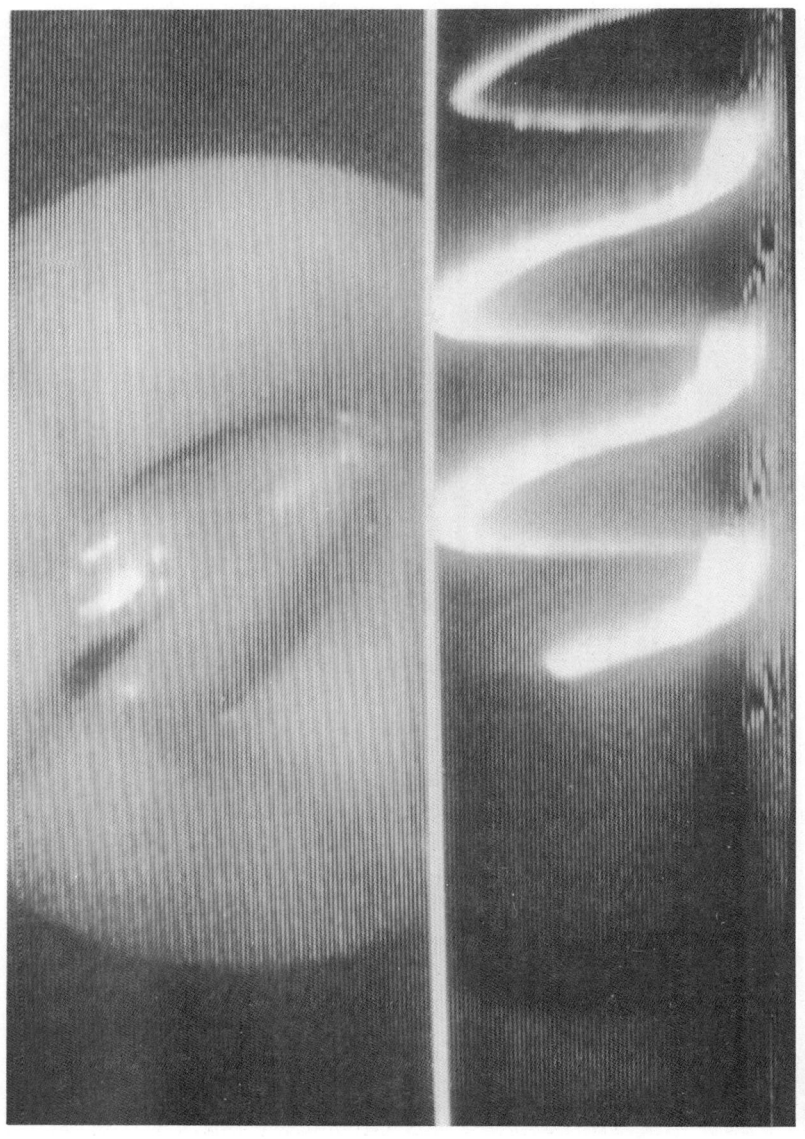

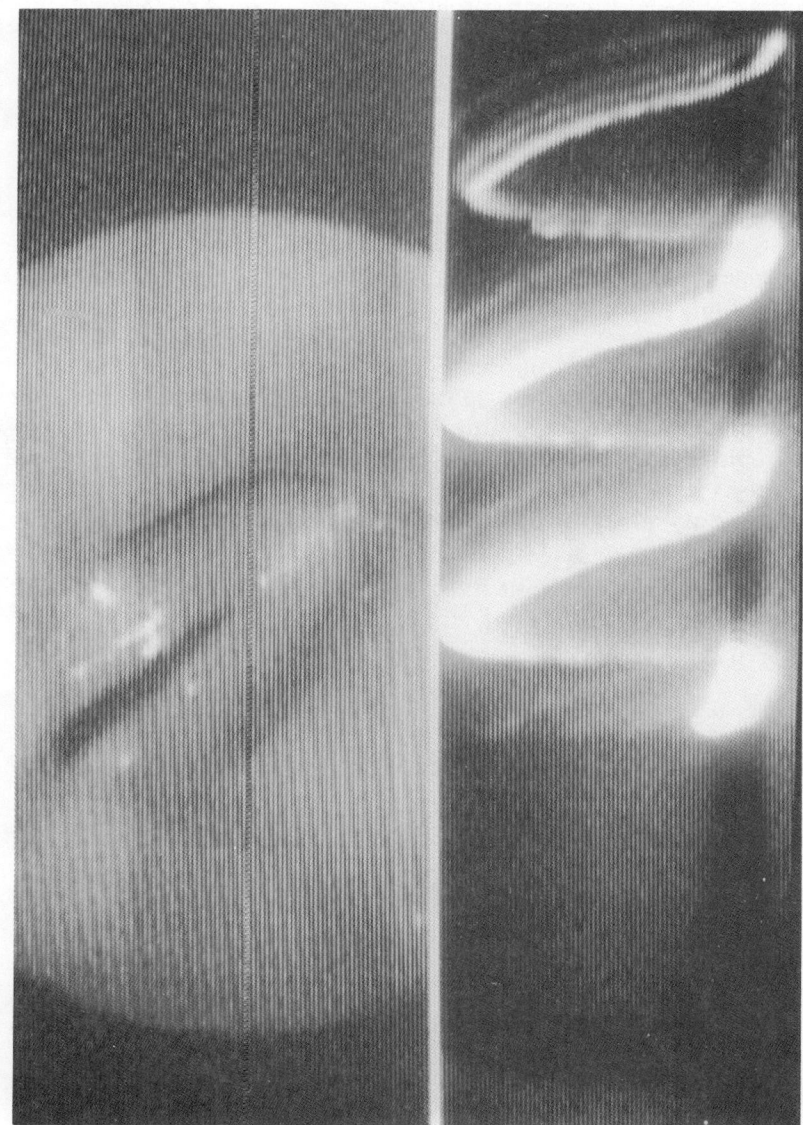

Figure 7-4. (continued)

In practice, the electroglottographic waveform appearing on the video monitor with the stroboscopic laryngeal image appears to move from right to left. This apparent movement is due to the stroboscopic triggering of the oscilloscopic display. The leading (far left) edge of the EGG waveform corresponds to the stroboscopic image. That point is referred to as the "trigger onset point." When the stroboscopic light flashes, an electrical signal is emitted from the light source to the oscilloscope which instantaneously sends the beam across the oscillographic display. The timing of the trigger onset point corresponds exactly with the timing of the stroboscopic light. In this manner, the position of the trigger onset point on the EGG waveform varies with the time during the glottal cycle when the stroboscopic light flashes. A resulting sequence of images is shown in Figure 7–4.

Synchronized videostroboscopy and electroglottography has been shown to be an effective tool for relating information from the electroglottographic waveform with information provided from stroboscopic images. For example, Karnell, Li, and Panje (1991) reported that the electroglottographic waveform can be useful for **confirming the time of maximum and minimum glottal closure** during voice production. A modified version of this approach has been included as an integral component of the recently introduced Kay Elemetrics stroboscopic system (Figure 7–5).

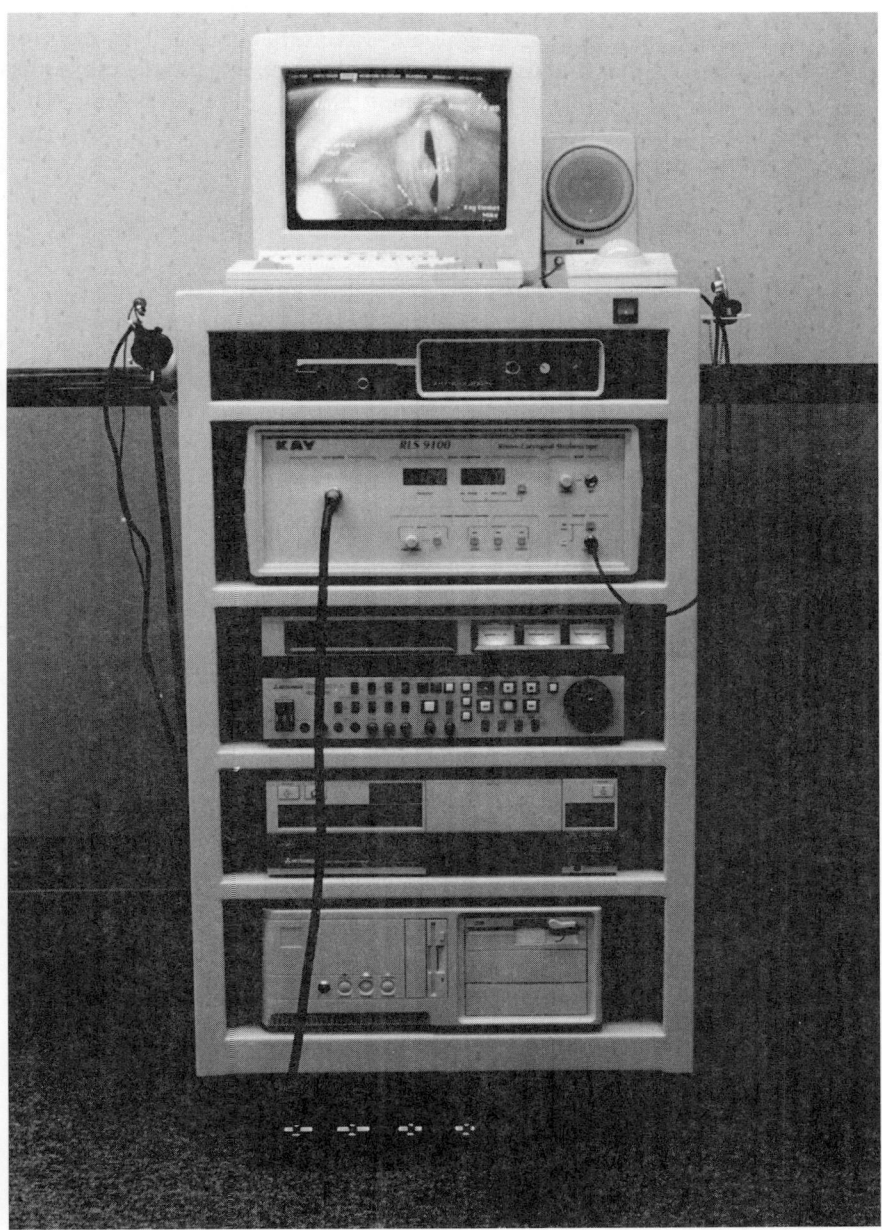

Figure 7–5. The Kay Elemetrics stroboscopic system includes synchronized electro-glottography and videostroboscopy as well as computer-supported videotape addressing and video printing capabilities.

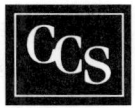

CHAPTER

8

Data Management

Perhaps the most important aspect of videoendoscopic and stroboscopic evaluations involves how the information from an evaluation is recorded and subsequently reported. Although there has been some consideration of interpretation of videoendoscopic images, little attention has been paid in the literature to how endoscopic data may be stored, retrieved, and reported. Computer data base systems are available to facilitate these important aspects of the videoendoscopic/stroboscopic evaluation process. The system in place at the author's institution will be described here. That system is used for videoendoscopic evaluation of velopharyngeal function, videostroboscopic evaluation of voice, and videoendoscopic evaluation of swallowing.

I. VIDEOENDOSCOPIC EVALUATION OF VELOPHARYNGEAL FUNCTION

A. Data Entry

The videoendoscopic data base utilizes a data entry form that contains all of the variables to be stored regarding velopharyngeal closure (Figure 8–1). Generally, the variables in the form

VELOPHARYNGEAL VIDEOENDOSCOPY / VIDEOFLUOROSCOPY DATA ENTRY FORM

| UNIT # | 1234567 | EVAL. DATE | 10/17/91 | BIRTHDATE | 4/8/77 | AGE | 15 | SEX | f |

PATIENT NAME   Jane Doe   ATTENDING   Dr. Skillful

TAPE #   185

1. REASON FOR REFERRAL [3]   1 = SUSPECTED VPI, 2 = PREOP EVAL, 3 = POSTOP EVAL, 4 = SUSPECTED OBSTR., 5 = OTHER (DESCRIBE BELOW IN HISTORY NOTES).

2. PATIENT HISTORY

CRANIOFACIAL ANOMALY/ [5]   CANCER [ ]   MUSCULAR FUNCTION DISORDER [ ]

CLEFT PALATE

1 = submucous
2 = soft palate only
3 = hard and soft palate only
4 = right unilateral complete
5 = left unilateral complete
6 = bilateral complete
7 = CPI

1 = hard palate
2 = soft palate
3 = left phar wall
4 = right phar wall
5 = post phar wall
6 = left tonsilar area
7 = right tonsilar area
8 = other (see notes)

1 = cerebral palsey, 2 = multiple sclerosis, 3 = ALS,
4 = trauma, 5 = dysarthria, 6 = other (see notes)

HISTORY NOTES

Jane is now post-op revision pharyngoplasty performed in July, 1991. At that time, the previously dehissed left side of the pharyngoplasty was repaired and anterior nasal surgery was performed to improve her nasal airway.

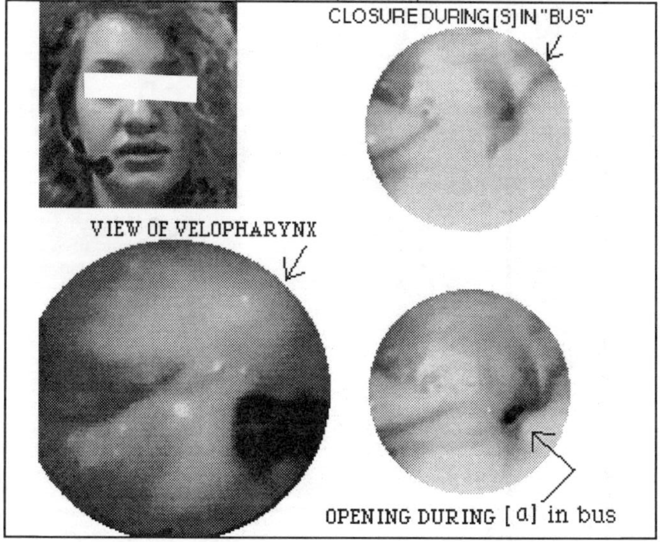

CLOSURE DURING [S]IN "BUS"

OPENING DURING [ɑ] in bus

VIEW OF VELOPHARYNX

144

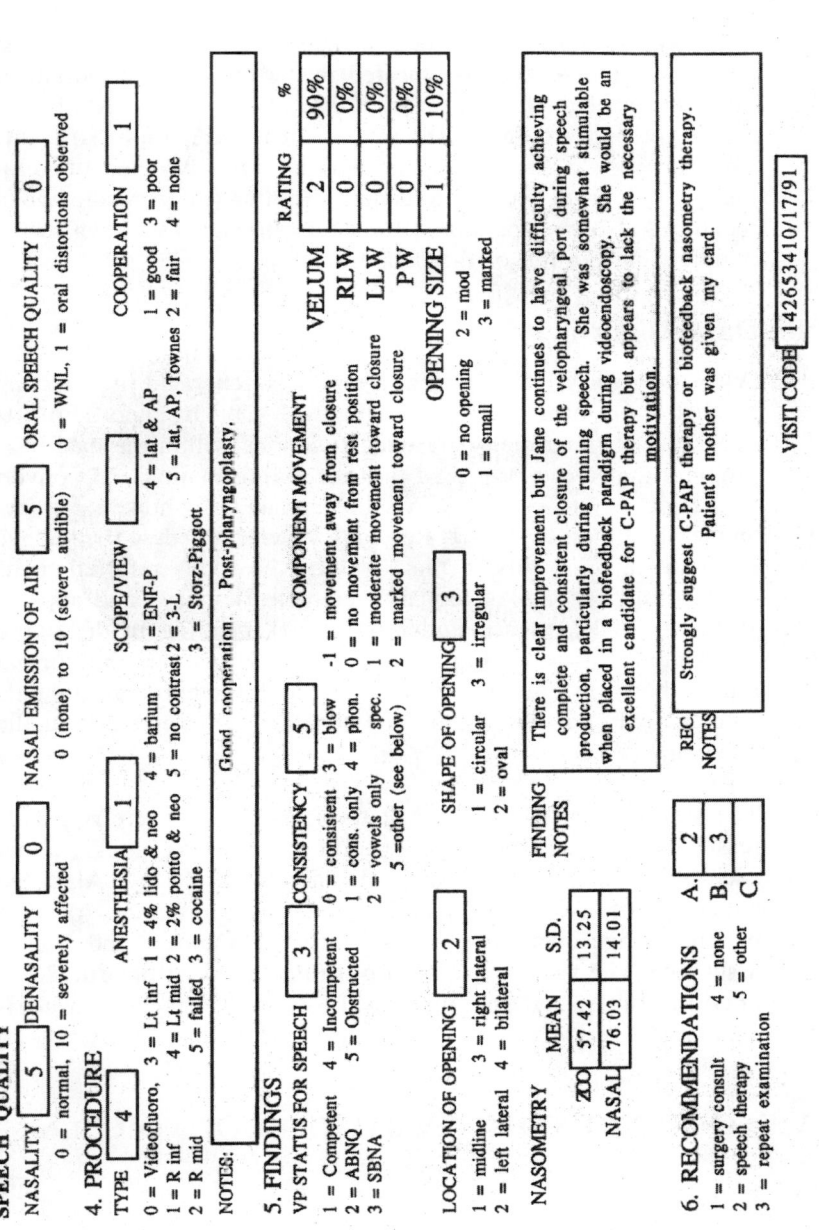

Figure 8-1. A computer-supported data base entry form for velopharyngeal videoendoscopic and videofluorographic data and images.

145

are standard observations typically obtained whenever videoendoscopic studies are performed. Most of the data entry fields are small and intended to accept few characters; in most cases just one. For example, the box located in the upper left quadrant of the form labeled "1. Reason for Referral" is used to record the reason for performing the study. The entry in Figure 8–1 for this variable was "1" indicating the patient was suspected of velopharyngeal insufficiency. Selected still images from the video recording also may be stored for later retrieval, as shown in the middle right portion of the data entry form.

B. Data Reporting

When data entry is completed, a report is generated by selecting another form labeled "Report" (Figure 8–2). The report form is generated from specially arranged functions within the data base program that locate and read the stored information and convert the single keystroke codes to sentences and/or phrases. For example, the "1" entry for "1. Reason for Referral," described above in Figure 8–1, results in the sentence "She was referred to us because of suspected velopharyngeal insufficiency" and appears as the second sentence under the report heading in the upper right-hand corner of Figure 8–2. In this manner, the formal report shown in Figure 8–2 is computer generated from the data entered in Figure 8–1, including the images selected from the videotape record.

The **standardized structure** of the report assists referring professionals who wish to locate specific information quickly about each aspect of resonance and velopharyngeal closure. Also, the data may be used subsequently for clinical research, tracking patient change over time, administrative accounting, and quality assurance. The system serves to **optimize clinical productivity, accountability,** and **reliability** while reducing demand on clerical support services.

II. VIDEOSTROBOSCOPIC EVALUATION OF VOICE

A. Data Entry

The videostroboscopic data base contains a data entry form that includes all the variables to be stored regarding laryngeal structure and vibratory activity (Figure 8–3). Generally, the variables in the form are standard observations typically obtained whenever video-strobscopic studies are performed (Hirano, 1984). Most of the data entry fields are small and intended to accept few characters; in most cases just one. For example, the box located in the upper left quadrant of the form labeled "G," for Grade of dysphonia, is used to record the patient's overall degree of perceived voice abnormality at the time of the study. The entry in Figure 8–3 for this variable was "2," indicating the patient was moderately dysphonic. Selected still images from the video recording may also be stored for later retrieval as shown in the middle right portion of the data entry form.

B. Data Reporting

When data entry is completed, a report is generated by selecting another form labeled "Report" (Figure 8–4). The report form is generated from specially arranged functions within the data base program that locate and read the stored information and convert the single keystroke codes to sentences and/or phrases. For example, the "2" entry for "Grade," described above, results in the sentence, "The patient's voice was moderately dysphonic," appearing as the first sentence under the "Perceived Voice Quality and Vocal Function" heading of the report. In this manner, the formal report shown in Figure 8–4 is computer generated from the data entered in Figure 8–3, including the images selected from the videotape record.

The advantages of the **standardized structure** of the report are similar to those summarized above regarding velopharyngeal examination data. Advantages regarding clinical research, tracking patient change over time, administrative accounting, quality assurance, and **optimizing clinical productivity, accountability, and reliability** are likewise similar.

III. DIGITAL IMAGE PROCESSING

Both data base systems described above incorporate digitized excerpts from the video record as data for storage and reporting. These images, produced from video hard copy devices, are frequently provided along with handwritten clinical notes describing the results of a study. It is very useful, however, to store images along with observations in

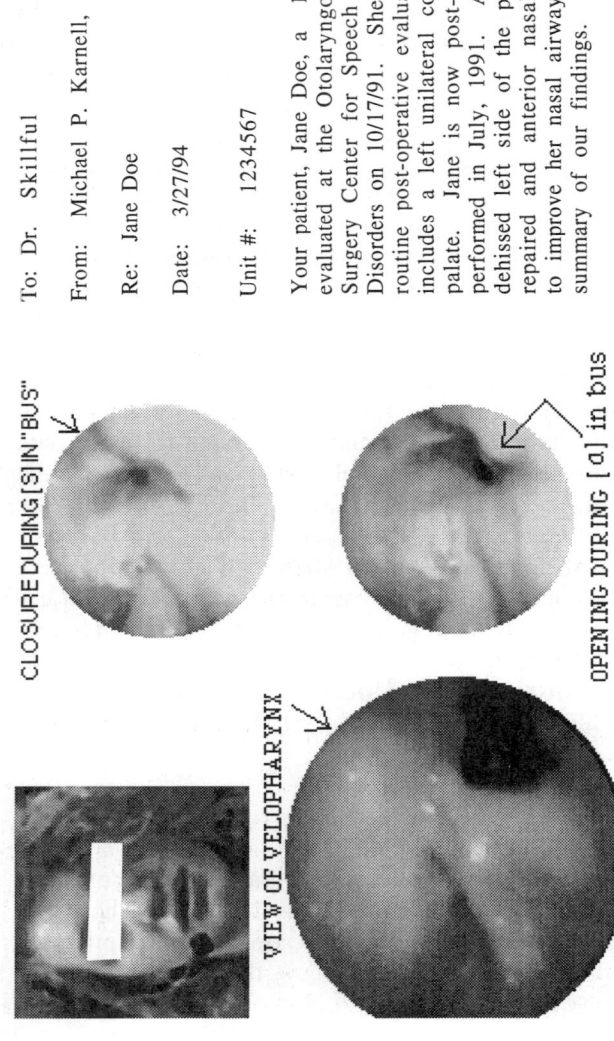

CLOSURE DURING [S] IN "BUS"

VIEW OF VELOPHARYNX

OPENING DURING [ɑ] in bus

To: Dr. Skillful

From: Michael P. Karnell, Ph.D.

Re: Jane Doe

Date: 3/27/94

Unit #: 1234567   Birthdate: 4/8/77

Your patient, Jane Doe, a 15 year old female, was evaluated at the Otolaryngology-Head and Neck Surgery Center for Speech and Swallowing Disorders on 10/17/91. She was referred to us for a routine post-operative evaluation. Her history includes a left unilateral complete cleft lip and palate. Jane is now post-op revision pharyngoplasty performed in July, 1991. At that time, the previously dehissed left side of the pharyngoplasty was repaired and anterior nasal surgery was performed to improve her nasal airway. The following is a summary of our findings.

PROCEDURES

Videoendoscopy was performed. A flexible fiberoptic endoscope was inserted through the patient's left middle nasal meatus. A 3.7 mm diameter scope was used. 4% lidocaine and 2% neosynephrine were applied prior to insertion. Patient cooperation was good. Post-pharyngoplasty.

SPEECH QUALITY

The patient's speech was hypernasal. Severity of hypernasality was judged as 5, where 0 = normal and 10 = severe. No hyponasality was noted. Audible nasal emission of air was observed. Severity of nasal emission was 5, where 0 = normal and 10 = severe. Oral speech quality was within normal limits. Average nasalance measured acoustically as the patient produced the zoo passage was 57.42 (greater than 32.0 is consistent with hypernasality). During production of standard nasal sentences, average nasalance was 76.03 (less than 50.0 is consistent with hyponasality).

VELOPHARYNGEAL PHYSIOLOGY

Marginal velopharyngeal insufficiency was observed. The patient achieved closure sometimes but not always. Inconsistent velopharyngeal closure was observed. Velar movement toward closure was marked, moving approximately 90% of the sagital port width. Right lateral pharyngeal wall movement toward closure was minimal, moving approximately 0% of the coronal port width. Left lateral pharyngeal wall movement toward closure was minimal, moving approximately 0% of the coronal port width. Posterior pharyngeal wall movement toward closure was minimal, moving approximately 0% of the sagital port width. At maximum velopharyngeal closure, a small opening, 10% of port size at rest, persisted. abnormal opening was visible to the left of midline. There is clear improvement but Jane continues to have difficulty achieving complete and consistent closure of the velopharyngeal port during speech production, particularly during running speech. She was somewhat stimulable when placed in a biofeedback paradigm during videoendoscopy. She would be an excellent candidate for C-PAP therapy but appears to lack the necessary motivation.

RECOMMENDATIONS

1. Speech therapy.

2. Repeat examination.

3.

NOTES

Strongly suggest C-PAP therapy or biofeedback nasometry therapy.
Patient's mother was given my card.

Figure 8–2. A computer-generated report automatically produced from the data in the entry form shown in Figure 8–1.

149

Laryngeal Videostroboscopy Data Entry Form

UNIT #	9876543
TAPE #	177
DATE	5/21/91

NAME Elaine Roe
ATTENDING Caring

BIRTHDATE 12/4/61
AGE (YEARS) 32
Report Date   Entry Date

G | 1 | 0 = NORM
R | 1 | 1 = MILD
B | 1 | 2 = MOD
A | 0 | 3 =
S | 0 | SEVERE

PITCH | 3 | 1 = NORM, 2 = HIGH, 3 = LOW
RANGE | 1 | 1 = NORM, 2 = RESTRICTED
BREAKS | 1 | 1 = NONE, 2 = > 1/SEC, 3 = < 1/SEC
RESP | 2 | 1 = IMPAIRED, 2 = NORM
Fo | 161 | IN HZ FROM STROBE

MPT 1 | 25 |
MPT 2 | |
MPT 3 | |
MEASURED IN SECONDS DURING SUSTAINED /a/

SCOPE | 3 |
1 = ENF P2
2 = RIGID 70
3 = BOTH

TYPE | 3 |
FAILED = 0 ENDO = 1
STROBE = 2
STROBE/EGG = 3

QUALITY | 2 |
EXC. = 1, GOOD = 2
FAIR = 3, POOR = 4

AMP. SYM | 1 |
AMP R | 1 |
AMP L | 1 |

SYM = 1, L>R = 2, R>L = 3
1 = NORMAL TO
5 = NO VISIBLE MOVEMENT

SUPRAGLOTTIC COMPRESSION | 1 |
1 = NONE TO 5 = SEVERE

PHASE SYM | 1 |
1 = NEVER IRREGULAR TO
5 = ALWAYS IRREGULAR

VOCAL FOLD EDGE RIGHT | 1 | LEFT | 1 |
1 (SMOOTH/STRAIGHT)
5 (ROUGH/IRREGULAR)

GLOTTAL CLOSURE | 1 |
COMPLETE = 1, INCONS. = 2
INCOMPLETE = 3

MUC. RIGHT | 1 |
WAVE LEFT | 1 |
Normal = 1
Small or absent = 2
Great = 3

OTHER OBS | 4 |
LONG. SULCUS = 1
WEBBING = 2
VENTR. HERNIA = 3
OTHER = 4 (describe)

DESCRIPTION
Evidence of hyperfunction. Edges of true folds pursed on adduction. Ventricular and arytenoid erytema.

150

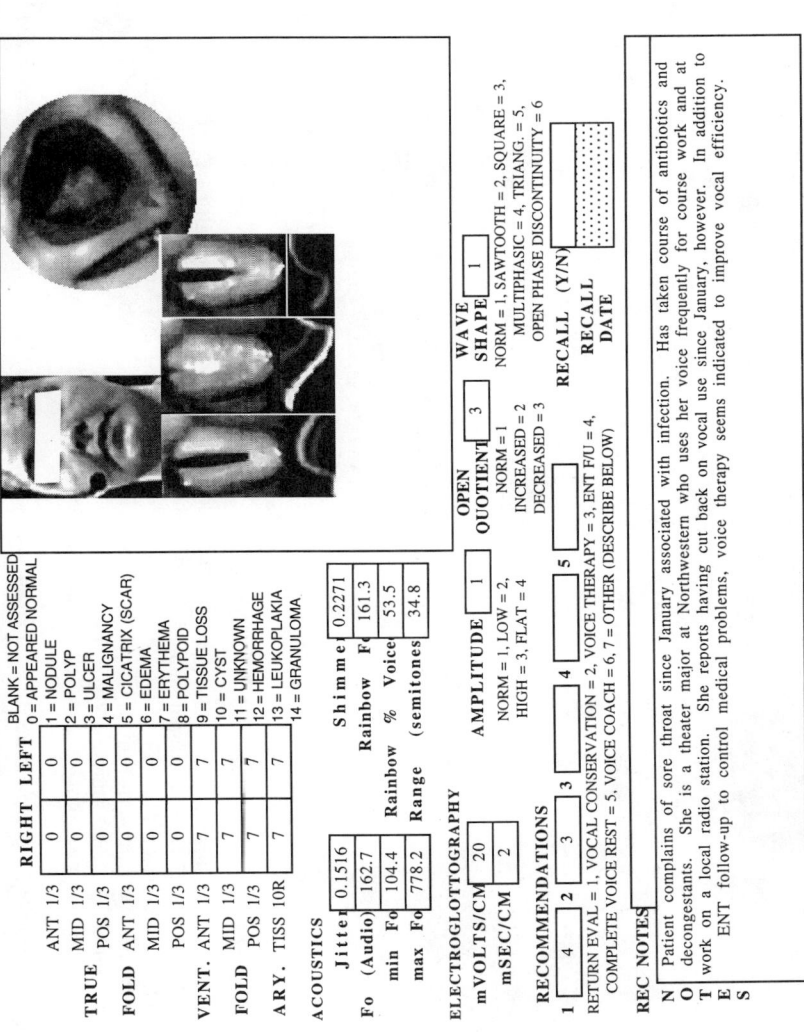

	RIGHT	LEFT	BLANK = NOT ASSESSED 0 = APPEARED NORMAL
ANT 1/3	0	0	1 = NODULE
TRUE MID 1/3	0	0	2 = POLYP
POS 1/3	0	0	3 = ULCER
FOLD ANT 1/3	0	0	4 = MALIGNANCY
MID 1/3	0	0	5 = CICATRIX (SCAR)
POS 1/3	0	0	6 = EDEMA
VENT. ANT 1/3	7	7	7 = ERYTHEMA
MID 1/3	7	7	8 = POLYPOID
FOLD POS 1/3	7	7	9 = TISSUE LOSS
ARY. TISS 10R	7	7	10 = CYST

11 = UNKNOWN
12 = HEMORRHAGE
13 = LEUKOPLAKIA
14 = GRANULOMA

ACOUSTICS

Jitter	0.1516		Shimmer	0.2271
Fo (Audio)	162.7		Rainbow Fo	161.3
min Fo	104.4		Rainbow % Voice	53.5
max Fo	778.2		Range (semitones)	34.8

ELECTROGLOTTOGRAPHY

mVOLTS/CM	20	AMPLITUDE	1	NORM = 1, LOW = 2, HIGH = 3, FLAT = 4
mSEC/CM	2			

OPEN QUOTIENT	3	NORM = 1 INCREASED = 2 DECREASED = 3

WAVE SHAPE	1	NORM = 1, SAWTOOTH = 2, SQUARE = 3, MULTIPHASIC = 4, TRIANG. = 5, OPEN PHASE DISCONTINUITY = 6

RECALL (Y/N)
RECALL DATE

RECOMMENDATIONS

| 1 | 4 | 2 | 3 | 3 | 4 | 4 | 5 |

RETURN EVAL = 1, VOCAL CONSERVATION = 2, VOICE THERAPY = 3, ENT F/U = 4,
COMPLETE VOICE REST = 5, VOICE COACH = 6, 7 = OTHER (DESCRIBE BELOW)

REC NOTES

N Patient complains of sore throat since January associated with infection. Has taken course of antibiotics and
O decongestants. She is a theater major at Northwestern who uses her voice frequently for course work and at
T work on a local radio station. She reports having cut back on vocal use since January, however. In addition to
E ENT follow-up to control medical problems, voice therapy seems indicated to improve vocal efficiency.
S

Figure 8–3. A computer-supported data base entry form for laryngeal videostroboscopic data and images.

The University of Iowa
Speech, Voice and Swallowing
Pathology

To: Dr. Caring

From: Michael P. Karnell, Ph.D.

Re: Elaine Roe

Date: 5/21/91 Unit # 9876543

Your patient, Ms. Roe, a 32 year old female, was evaluated at the Center for Speech and Swallowing Disorders on 5/21/91. The following is a summary of our findings.

Perceived Voice Quality and Vocal Function

The patient's voice quality was mildly dysphonic. Voice quality was characterized by mild roughness, mild breathiness, no asthenia, and no strained quality. Perceived habitual pitch was judged to be abnormally low, given the patient's age and gender. Vocal pitch range was judged to be within normal limits. Pitch breaks were not observed during the evaluation. Measured fundamental frequency during habitual pitch production was 162.7 Hz. Maximum phonation time was 25 seconds (minimum for children = 15 sec., for women = 20 sec., for men = 25 sec). Mean relative pitch perturbation (jitter) was 0.1516%. Mean relative amplitude perturbation (shimmer) was 0.2271%.

Physiologic Observations

Videostroboscopy with synchronized electroglottography (EGG) was performed. The quality of the video record was good. The medial edge of the vocal folds appeared smooth and straight on the right and appeared smooth and straight on the left. No supraglottic compression was observed. Glottal closure was consistently complete. Amplitude of vocal fold movement was symmetrical. Amplitude of right vocal fold movement was within normal limits. Amplitude of left vocal fold movement was within normal limits. Vocal fold vibration was consistently symmetrical. The right vocal fold mucosal wave was within normal limits. The left vocal fold mucosal wave was within normal limits.

Evidence of hyperfunction. Edges of true folds pursed on adduction. Ventricular and arytenoid erytema.

Laryngeal Tissue Observations*

	RIGHT SIDE	LEFT SIDE
A. Anterior 1/3 of medial edge of true fold	Normal	Normal
B. Middle 1/3 of medial edge of true fold	Normal	Normal
C. Posterior 1/3 of medial edge of true fold	Normal	Normal
D. Anterior 1/3 of superior surface of true fold	Normal	Normal
E. Middle 1/3 of superior surface of true fold	Normal	Normal
F. Posterior 1/3 of superior surface of true fold	Normal	Normal
G. Anterior 1/3 of ventricular fold	Erythema	Erythema
H. Middle 1/3 of ventricular fold	Erythema	Erythema
I. Posterior 1/3 of ventricular told	Erythema	Erythema
J. Posterior commissure and/or arytenoid	Erythema	Erythema

* Tissue changes reported here are not exclusive and are subject to medical confirmation.

Electroglottographic (EGG) Assessment of Vocal Fold Contact

EGG waveform amplitude was normal indicating normal vocal fold contact. The shape of the EGG waveform was within normal limits. EGG open quotient appeared reduced, suggesting increased duration of vocal fold contact.

Additional Notes and Comments

Patient complains of sore throat since January associated with infection. Has taken course of antibiotics and decongestants. She is a theater major at Northwestern who uses her voice frequently for course work and at work on a local radio station. She reports having cut back on vocal use since January, however. In addition to ENT follow-up to control medical problems, voice therapy seems indicated to improve vocal efficiency.

Recommendations

1. ENT follow-up.   2. Voice Therapy.

Figure 8–4. A computer-generated report automatically produced from the data in the entry form shown in Figure 8–3.

the computer data base. The process of **acquiring, enhancing,** and **storing** these images in the data base system will be described here.

Still images may be **extracted from the videotape record** by using commercially available video digitizing boards coupled with a desktop computer. The purpose of the digitizing board is to convert video images into a numerical form that can be manipulated and stored on the computer. Software for controlling the board and manipulating the images is frequently provided when the board is purchased. Other programs are available for this purpose also.

The system described above included a Data Translation "Quick-Capture" digitizing board mounted on a Macintosh computer, the same computer that is used to run the data base program described previously. The software used to control the board and enhance the captured images is entitled "Image" (Wayne Rasband, National Institutes of Health). A cable connecting the "video out" port on the back of the VCR and the video digitizing board provides the means of transferring the image from the VCR to the computer.

To digitize, or "capture" an image, the "Image" software program is initiated. The videotape is cued to display the desired video image on the video monitor. The program is then set for "capture," and the image that appears on the VCR monitor simultaneously appears on the computer monitor. The user then turns off the "capture" mode, and the image remains stored in the computer's memory and continues to appear on the computer screen.

The images provided are usually larger than are useful for data base management and reporting. They may also be darker than desired. The "Image" program is used to **reduce, brighten,** and/or **sharpen** the contrast of the portion of the image that is to be stored. Images acquired via nasal videoendoscopy frequently appear rotated on the videotape record, because the flexible endoscope is frequently rotated somewhat during the procedure in order to obtain the best possible image of the velopharyngeal or laryngeal structures. The program can be used to **rotate** these images so that the orientation of structures is more easily interpreted.

Groups of images may be acquired and assembled as components of a single composite image that is then **stored with the clinical observations.** These components usually include a picture of the patient's face and several pictures of the velopharynx or larynx at specific points during a speech or voice gesture. Text may be added to the images along with arrows to facilitate interpretation. The composite image is copied into memory and stored as image data in the data base program described above.

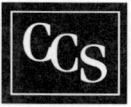

CHAPTER

9

Training

A s stated earlier, formal opportunities for learning videoendoscopic/stroboscopic procedures and techniques are few. There are occasional short courses and seminars on the topic offered at professional meetings, but they rarely provide hands-on experience. Actual experience with endoscopy has been limited to that which takes place in the clinical setting itself. A colleague (Riski, personal communication) recently commented about how otolaryngologists are typically trained to performed endoscopy as follows:

> . . . They have a "time honored" tradition of giving a resident a patient and an endoscope with the purpose of evaluating the vocal tract. I don't think their training goes much beyond that.

This is consistent with the author's experience at two large, well-known, academic medical centers. Residents appear to learn by **clinical observation, trial and error**. Many residents who perform endoscopy have never had it performed on themselves and, therefore, have little basis for empathizing with the patient's point of view. Undeniably, they seem to learn the procedure and perform it routinely with some apparent success. Little can be said about the adequacy of the endoscopic studies performed, because there is usually little formal documentation and no means by which to assure quality. The addition of video recording should be helpful in these areas if video is used routinely.

Given the rather informal, yet successful, "training" tradition described above, and the fact that videoendoscopy is a diagnostic procedure and not a formal area of academic inquiry, it may seem excessive to consider the need for formal training, particularly for medical students and residents. Speech pathologists, however, should be more careful and deliberate in their attempts to become competent with the procedure (ASHA, 1992).

There is need to develop **minimal levels of observation, hands-on instruction, and actual clinical experience** with the procedure for speech pathologists interested in becoming endoscopically competent. Table 9–1 contains some proposed **objectives** that a workshop on endoscopy should achieve. This course should ensure that attendees acquire a basic level of understanding of why and how the procedure is performed; provide experience performing the procedure in a controlled environment; and, perhaps most importantly, provide opportunity for interpretation and discussion of completed studies. Instruction should also cover report writing and record keeping.

The **extent** and **cost** of videoendoscopy training must be consistent with the complexity and risks involved. Initial training can be obtained in a well structured workshop over the course of 3–4 days. The outline provided in Table 9–2 should enable the speech pathologist with special interest and academic preparation in anatomy and physiology of speech and voice production to acquire the

Table 9–1. Proposed objectives for a workshop designed to offer a minimal level of training in videoendoscopy/stroboscopy

1. To familiarize attendee(s) with the rationale for videoendoscopic and stroboscopic assessment of velopharyngeal and laryngeal function for speech production.

2. To provide experience managing equipment involved with videoendoscopic and stroboscopic assessment of velopharyngeal and laryngeal function for speech production.

3. To provide experience performing videoendoscopic and stroboscopic assessment of velopharyngeal and laryngeal function for speech production.

4. To provide experience in the interpretation and reporting of results of videoendoscopic and stroboscopic assessment of velopharyngeal and laryngeal function for speech production.

Table 9–2. Outline of a proposed three-day workshop designed to provide training in videoendoscopy/stroboscopy

Morning Session
   I. Course overview (15 min)
  II. Role of videoendoscopy/stroboscopy in the Clinical Process (30 min)
 III. Types of videoendoscopy/stroboscopy (15 min)
 IV. Tour of clinical laboratory (30 min)
  V. Supporting measures (30 min)
     A. Perceptual measures
     B. Acoustic measures
 VI. Patient Videotape Review (45 min)
VII. Discussion (15 min)

Afternoon Session
   I. Introduction to patient management. (30 min)
  II. Introduction to technique and interpretation (90 min)
     A. Rigid scope, oral insertion
     B. Rigid scope, laryngeal views
     B. Flexible scope, nasal insertion
     C. Flexible scope, velopharyngeal views
     D. Flexible scope, pharyngeal/laryngeal views
 III. Patient Videotape Review (45 min)
 IV. Discussion (15 min)

Morning Session
   I. Video recording equipment management and care (30 min)
  II. Endoscope management and care (30 min)
 III. Introduction to scope insertion (45 min)
 IV. Patient observation (60 min)
  V. Discussion (15 min)

Afternoon Session
   I. Scope insertion practice (60 min)
  II. Patient observation (60 min)
 III. Interpretation—Patient Videotape Review (45 min)
 IV. Discussion (15)

Morning Session
   I. Scope insertion practice (60 min)
  II. Patient observation (60 min)
 III. Interpretation—Patient Videotape Review (45 min)
 IV. Discussion

Afternoon Session
   I. Scope insertion practice (60 min)
  II. Patient observation (60 min)
 III. Image analysis and data base management (30 min)
 IV. Discussion (30 min)

minimal level of training in videoendoscopy/stroboscopy needed to get started. This outline provides for a total of 4 hours of lecture presentation regarding equipment, procedures, and reporting techniques; 4 hours of videotape review and discussion; 4 hours of patient observation; and 3 hours of hands-on experience with the endoscope. This amount of exposure and experience should enable the student to begin to perform the procedure under the supervision of experienced endoscopists within the supportive environment of the clinic. *The experience gained from months of hands-on experience with patients cannot be duplicated in a workshop.* The workshop can, however, provide the necessary foundation of knowledge and experience that would make more extensive experience possible.

Training in performing videoendoscopy may not provide in-depth knowledge about the subtleties of velopharyngeal closure or laryngeal vibratory behavior in the variety of patients evaluated in the clinic. **Graduate level coursework** in cleft palate, voice disorders, speech production, swallowing disorders, and related educational experiences should provide the basic information needed in these areas. The highly specialized information provided in professional seminars and symposia is invaluable to the developing endoscopist. The value of continuing education for those interested in using videoendoscopy to evaluate voice, resonance, and swallowing disorders cannot be overstated.

Academic programs that are not located within a medical complex cannot support nasal videoendoscopy training. As stated previously, nasal insertion of the flexible endoscope, although generally safe, places the patient at some risk for nasal trauma and unexpected allergic reaction to anesthesia. For this reason, **nasal videoendoscopic training should be provided only in a medical center**. Oral endoscopic training and experience may be provided in the typical speech-language pathology and audiology academic facility, provided adequate consideration is given to safety, cleanliness, ethical issues, and insurance coverage.

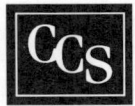

REFERENCES

Anastaplo, S., & Karnell, M. P. (1988). Synchronized videostroboscopic and electro-glottographic examination of glottal opening. *Journal of the Acoustical Society of America, 83*, 1883–1890.

American Speech-Language-Hearing Association. (1992). Vocal tract visualization and imaging. *Asha, 34* (March Suppl. 7), 37–40.

Bastian, R. W., & Nagorsky, M. J. (1987). Laryngeal image biofeedback. *Laryngoscope, 97*, 1346–1349.

Bless, D. (1987). Stroboscopic evaluation of the larynx. *Training seminar on videostroboscopy for laryngologists/speech pathologists.* Chicago: Bruel & Kjäer.

CDC. (1989). Guidelines for prevention of transmission of human immunodeficiency virus and hepatitis B virus in health-care and public-safety workers. *MMWR, 38*, No. S-6.

Covello, L., Karnell, M. P., & Seaver, E. J. (1992). Videoendoscopy and photodetection: Linearity of a new integrated system. *Cleft Palate-Craniofacial Journal, 29*, 168–173.

Dalston, R. M. (1982). Photodetection assessment of velopharyngeal activity. *Cleft Palate Journal, 19.* 1–8.

Dalston, R. M. (1989). Using simultaneous photodetection and nasometry to monitor velopharyngeal behavior during speech. *Journal of Speech and Hearing Research, 32*, 195–202.

Dalston, R. M., & Seaver, E. J. (1990). Nasometric and phototransductive measurements of reaction times among normal adult speakers. *Cleft Palate Journal, 27*, 61–67.

Dixon, H. S. (1992). Allergy and laryngeal disease. *Otolaryngologic Clinics of North America. 25*(1), 239–250.

Ford, C. N., Bless, D. M., & Lowery, J. D. (1990). Indirect laryngoscopic approach for injection of botulinum toxin in spasmodic dysphonia. *Otolaryngology—Head and Neck Surgery. 103*(5, Pt 1), 752–758.

Golding-Kushner, K. J., Argamaso, R. V., Cotton, R. T., Grames, L. M., Henningsson, G., Jones, D. L., Karnell, M. P., Klaiman, P. G., Lewin, M. L., Marsh, J. L., McCall, G. N., McGrath, C. O., Muntz, H. R., Nevdahl, M. T., Rakoff, S. J., Shprintzen, R. J., Sidoti, E. J., Vallino, L. D., Volk, M., Williams, W. N., Witzel, M. A., Dixon Wood, V. L., Ysunza, A., D'Antonio, L., Isberg, A., Pigott, R. W., & Skolnick, L. (1990). Standardization for the reporting of nasopharyngoscopy and multiview videofluoroscopy: A report from an international working group. *Cleft Palate Journal, 27*, 337–347.

Grundfast, K. M., & Harley, E. (1989). Vocal cord paralysis. *Otolaryngologic Clinics of North America. 22*(3), 569–597.

Hacki, T., Kenklies, M., Hofmann, R., & Haferkamp, G. (1990). Pharmakotherapie von Stimm- und Artikulationsstörungen bei Aphasie. *Folia Phoniatrica, 42*(6), 283–288.

Hirano, M. (1984). *Clinical examination of voice.* New York: Springer-Verlag.

Hirano, M., Bless, D. M. (1993). *Videostroboscopic examination of the larynx.* San Diego: Singular Publishing Group.

Hynes, W. (1950). Pharyngoplasty by muscle transplantation. *British Journal of Plastic Surgery, 3*, 138.

Ibuki, K., Karnell, M. P., & Morris, H. L. (1983). The nasopharyngeal fiberscope for assessing velopharyngeal function: Reliability and validity of analysis by measurement. *Cleft Palate Journal, 20*, 97–104.

Ibuki, K., Morris, H. L., Miyazaki, T., Matsuya, T., & Karnell, M. P. (1982). Reliability and validity of nasopharyngeal fiberscopic (NPF) examination: A simultaneous NPF and lateral cinefluoroscopic (Cine) study. *Journal of the Japanese Cleft Palate Association, 7*, 29–47.

Jackson, I. T. (1985). Sphincter pharyngoplasty. In W. C. Trier, (Ed.), *Clinics in plastic surgery* (pp. 711–718). Philadelphia: W. B. Saunders Co.

Karnell, M. P. (1983). The nasopharyngeal fiber-scope. [Letter to the Editor] *Cleft Palate Journal, 20*, 260–261.

Karnell, M. P. (1989). Synchronized videostroboscopy and electroglottography. *Journal of Voice, 3*, 68–75.

Karnell, M. P., Ibuki, K., Morris, H. L., & Van Demark, D. R. (1983). The nasopharyngeal fiberscope for assessing velopharyngeal function: Reliability and validity of analysis by judgment. *Cleft Palate Journal, 20*, 199–208.

Karnell, M. P., Isdebski, K., Morris, H., Stone, R. E., Waterson, T., Wilson, F. B., & Witzell, M. A. (1992, November). Nasal videoendoscopy: *Issues in Training and Ethics.* Miniseminar presented at the Annual Meeting of the American Speech-Language-Hearing Association, San Antonio.

Karnell, M. P., Li, L., & Panje, W. R. (1991). Glottal opening in patients with vocal fold tissue changes. *Journal of Voice, 5*, 239–246.

Karnell, M. P., Linville, R. N., & Edwards, B. A. (1988). Variations in velar position over time: A nasal endoscopic study. *Journal of Speech and Hearing Research, 31*, 417–424.

Karnell, M. P., & Morris, H. L. (1985). Multiview videoendoscopic evaluation of velopharyngeal physiology in fifteen normal speakers. *Annals of Otology, Rhinology, and Laryngology, 94*, 361–365.

Karnell, M. P., & Seaver, E. J. (1993). A new integrated videoendoscopy-photodetector system for assessment of velopharyngeal insufficiency. *Cleft Palate-Craniofacial Journal*, *30*, 337–342.

Karnell, M. P., Seaver, E. J., & Dalston, R. M. (1988). A comparison of photodetector and endoscopic evaluations of velopharyngeal function. *Journal of Speech and Hearing Research*, *31*, 503–510.

Keefe, M. J., & Dalston, R. M. (1989). An analysis of velopharyngeal timing in normal adult speakers using a microcomputer based photodetector system. *Journal of Speech and Hearing Research*, *32*, 39–48.

Kitzing, P. (1985). Stroboscopy—A pertinent laryngological examination. *The Journal of Otolaryngology*, *14*(3), 151–157.

Kruse, E. (1989). Differential diagnosis of functional voice disorders. *Folia Phoniatrica*, *41*(1), 1–9.

Kunzel, H. J. (1982). First applications of a biofeedback device for the therapy of velopharyngeal incompetence. *Folia Phoniatrica*, *34*, 92–100.

Langmore, S. E., Schatz, K., & Olsen, N. (1988). Fiberoptic endoscopic examination of swallowing safety: A new procedure. *Dysphagia*, *2*, 216–219.

Linville, S. E. (1992). Glottal gap configurations in two age groups of women. *Journal of Speech and Hearing Research*, *35*, 1209–1215.

Logemann, J. A. (1983). *Evaluation and treatment of swallowing disorders*. San Diego: College-Hill Press.

Moeller, D. (1976). *Speech pathology and audiology: Iowa origins of a discipline*. Iowa City: The University of Iowa Press.

Morris, H. L. (1984). Marginal velopharyngeal incompetence. In H. Winitz (Ed.), *Treating articulation disorders: For clinicians by clinicians*. Baltimore: University Park Press.

Orticochea, M. (1968). Construction of a dynamic muscle sphincter in cleft palates. *Journal of Plastic and Reconstructive Surgery*, *41*, 323.

Pigott, R. W. (1969). The nasendoscopic appearance of the normal palato-pharyngeal valve. *Journal of Plastic and Reconstructive Surgery*, *43*, 19–24.

Pluzhnikov, M. S., Lopatko, A. I., & Ibrakhem, M. (1992). Laser surgery and phototherapy of the larynx and laryngopharynx under indirect laryngoscopy. *Vestnik Oto-Rino-Laringologii*, *1*, 20–24.

Ptok, M. (1993). Pseudoglottis after laryngeal trauma with bilateral recurrent laryngeal nerve paralysis. *HNO*, *41*(1), 41–46.

Riski, J. E., Ruff, G. L., Georgiade, G. S., Barwick, W. J., & Edwards, P. D. (1992). Evaluation of sphincter pharyngoplasty. *Cleft Palate Journal*, *29*, 254–261.

Sataloff, R. T. (1991). *Professional voice: The science and art of clinical care*. New York: Raven Press.

Sataloff, R.T., Spiegel J. R., & Hawkshaw, M. J. (1991). Strobovideolaryngoscopy: Results and clinical value. *Annals of Otology, Rhinology and Laryngology*, *100*(9, Pt. 1), 725–727.

Sercarz, J. A., Berke, G. S., Ming, Y., & Gerratt, B. R. (1992). Videostroboscopy of human vocal fold paralysis. *Annals of Otology, Rhinology and Laryngology*, *101*(7), 567–577.

Shprintzen, R. J. (1983). An invited commentary on the preceding article by Ibuki, Karnell and Morris. *Cleft Palate Journal*, *20*, 105-107.

Shprintzen, R. J., Lewin, M. L., Croft, C. B., Daniller, A. I., Argamaso, R. V., Ship, A.

G., & Strauch, B. (1979). A comprehensive study of pharyngeal flap surgery: Tailor made flaps. *Cleft Palate Journal, 16*(1), 46–55.

Siegel-Sadewitz, V. L., & Shprintzen, R. J. (1982). Nasopharyngoscopy of the normal velopharyngeal sphincter: An experiment of biofeedback. *Cleft Palate Journal, 19*, 194–200.

Slavit, D. H., & Maragos, N. E. (1992). Physiologic assessment of arytenoid adduction. *Annals of Otology, Rhinology and Laryngology, 101*(4), 321–327.

Smith, R. M. (1980). *Anesthesia for infants and children* (4th ed.). St. Louis: C.V. Mosby Co.

Sodersten, M., & Lindestad, P. A. (1992). A comparison of vocal fold closure in rigid telescopic and flexible fiberoptic laryngostroboscopy. *Acta Otolaryngologica (Stockholm), 112*, 144–150.

Taub, S. (1966). The Taub oral panendoscope: A new technique. *Cleft Palate Journal, 3*, 328–346.

von Leden, H., Moore, P., & Timcke, R. (1960). Laryngeal vibrations: Measurements of the glottic wave. Part III: The pathologic larynx. *Archives of Otolaryngology, 71*, 26–45.

Wallesch, B., Sieron, J., & Johannsen, H. S. (1991). The value of indirect microlaryngo-stroboscopy in the follow-up care of patients with vocal cord carcinoma treated with primary irradiation. *Laryngo-Rhino-Otologie. 70*(10), 559–561.

Watterson, T., McFarlane, S. C., & Menicucci, A. L. (1990). Vibratory characteristics of teflon-injected and noninjected paralyzed vocal folds. *Journal of Speech and Hearing Disorders, 55*, 61–66.

Willis, C. R., & Stutz, M. L. (1972). The clinical use of the Taub oral panendoscope in the observation of velopharyngeal function. *Journal of Speech and Hearing Research, 37*, 495–502.

Yanagisawa, E., & Yanagisawa, K. (1993). Stroboscopic videolaryngoscopy: A comparison of fiberscopic and telescopic documentation. *Annals of Otology, Rhinology and Laryngology, 102*, 255–265.

Zhao, R. (1992). Diagnostic value of stroboscopy in early glottic carcinoma. *Chung Hua Erh Pi Yen Hou Ko Tsa Chih* [Chinese Journal of Otorhinolaryngology], *27*(3), 175–176, 191.

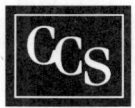

APPENDIX

A

A Review of Universal Precautions Applied to Videoendoscopy

All health care professionals who clinically manage patients should be aware of the Center for Disease Control's guidelines for prevention of transmission of serious infectious diseases like human immunodeficiency virus (HIV) and hepatitis B (CDC, 1989). Clinicians who perform videoendoscopy may be, by the nature of the procedure, exposed to body fluids that may carry these infectious diseases. It is essential, therefore, that those clinicians take the necessary precautions to protect themselves and their patients from infectious diseases that may be transmitted during the videoendoscopic examination.

The term *Universal Precautions* refers to the assumption that any patient may have unrecognized infection with HIV or other infectious agents transmissible by blood or other body fluids. The precautions against transmission of these disease agents must, therefore, be applied universally (i.e., to *all* patients). With regard to videoendoscopy, universal precautions include consideration of barriers against infection as well as cleaning procedures. Prevention of injuries caused by needles, scalpels, and other sharp instruments is not an issue for videoendoscopy because no sharp objects are needed or used. Special procedures regarding the handling of patients with known infections are usually required. The clinician performing endoscopy should consult with medical personnel regarding the specifics of handling patients with known infectious diseases.

I. BARRIERS

Spread of infection can be prevented, in part, by the use of protective barriers that prevent contact with potentially infectious body fluids. There is need for two types of barriers when performing videoendoscopy: gloves and protective eyeglasses.

A. Gloves

Nonsterile rubber gloves should be worn any time that an endoscope is handled. Sterile gloves are not necessary because no body incisions are made which would require maintenance of a sterile field for protection of the patient. Nonsterile gloves provide adequate protection for the patient while preventing contact between the clinician's hands and the patient's saliva or other mucous secretions that might be otherwise contacted when handling the endoscope or performing manual tongue anchoring procedures. Rubber gloves should be disposed of immediately after use with each patient.

B. Protective Eyeglasses

Eye barriers are important given the possibility that the endoscopic procedure may stimulate a sneeze, cough, or gag reflex from the patient resulting in airborne transmission of potentially infected saliva and mucus that could otherwise strike the exposed clinician's eyes.

II. CLEANING PROCEDURES

The importance of well structured cleaning procedures for the clinician's hands and the endoscopes to be used cannot be overstated. The clinician's hands must be cleaned thoroughly with soap and water before and after performing a procedure even when using gloves.

Minor skin lesions on the clinician's hands must be cleaned, covered with a dressing, and protected with gloves. Clinicians with weeping dermatitis or exudative skin lesions on their hands should refrain from all direct patient care and from handling patient care equipment until the condition resolves. For routine handwashing, a rigorous rubbing of all surfaces of lathered hands, for at least 10 seconds, followed by a thorough rinsing is recommended.

The endoscopes and atomizers (used for application of topical anesthetics and vasoconstrictors) should be thoroughly washed with soap and water immediately following each use. Personnel performing endoscopic cleaning procedures should wear disposable protective gloves. The endoscope surfaces should be cleaned thoroughly with soap and water and dried with a clean disposable towel. The endoscope insertion tube should then be wiped clean with a 1:100 dilution of bleach or 70% isopropyl alcohol or soaked for a minimum of 45 minutes in 2% glutaraldehyde (e.g., Cidex®) or comparable chemical to ensure 100% kill of microorganisms including **Mycobacterium tuberculosis**.[1] After soaking, the instrument should be dried with a clean disposable cloth and stored in its case. The storage case should never be contaminated with a soiled endoscope. Surfaces that may have been soiled by patient saliva or mucus via coughing or sneezing should be wiped clean with a 1:100 dilution of bleach or 70% isopropyl alcohol. Gloves worn by personnel performing the cleaning procedures must be disposed of immediately and the hands must be washed after the gloves have been removed.

---

[1] The specifics of these procedures may vary somewhat across institutions. The clinician should be familiar with the guidelines in place at the institution where the procedure is to be performed.

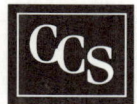

APPENDIX

B

Videoendoscopy Component Vendors

The following are the major vendors of various videoendoscopic or videostroboscopic components. A listing here is not intended to imply endorsement, nor is absence from this list intended to imply lack of endorsement.

Bruel & Kjäer
This company was a major vendor of videostroboscopic components in the 1980s (see Figure 3–4, page 33) but currently does not offer videostroboscopic equipment.

Karl Storz Endoscopy of
  America, Inc.
600 Corporate Point
Culver City, CA 90230-7600
Information: 310-558-1500
Toll Free: 800-421-0837

FAX: 800-321-1304
Offer:
  rigid endoscopes
  endoscopic light sources
  video cameras
  video recorders
  video printers
  video monitors
  image managmeent systems

Kay Elemetrics Corp.
12 Maple Ave.
Pine Brook, NJ 07058

Toll Free: 800-289-5297
FAX: 201-227-7760
Offer:
  rigid laryngeal endoscopes
  stroboscopic light sources
  video cameras
  video recorders
  video printers
  video monitors
  image management systems

Machida Endoscopes
Smith and Nephew Richards,
  Distributor
1450 Brooks Road
Memphis, TN 38116
Toll Free: 800-238-7538
FAX: 910-373-0220
Offer:
  flexible endoscopes
  endoscopic light sources
  video cameras
  video recorders
  video printers
  video monitors
  image management systems

Nagashima Instruments
Kelleher Medical, Inc.
9710 Farrar Court, Suite N
Richmond, VA 23236
Information: 804-323-4040
FAX: 804-323-4073
Offer:
  rigid laryngeal endoscopes
  stroboscopic light sources
  video cameras
  video recorders
  video printers
  video monitors
  image management systems

Olympus Corporation of America
4 Nevada Drive
Lake Success, NY 11042
Information: 516-488-3880
Toll Free: 800-645-8160
FAX: 516-326-9085
Offer:
  flexible endoscopes
  endoscopic light sources
  video cameras
  video recorders
  video printers
  video monitors
  image management systems

Pentax Precision Instrument
  Company
30 Ramland Road
Orangeburg, NY 10962-2699
Information: 914-365-0700
Toll Free: 800-431-5880
FAX: 914-365-0822
Offer:
  flexible endoscopes
  endoscopic light sources
  video cameras
  video recorders
  video printers
  video monitors
  image management systems

Wolf Instruments
Richard Wolf Medical Instruments
  Corporation
353 Corporate Woods Parkway
Vernon Hills, IL 60061
Information: 708-913-1113
Toll Free (Ordering only): 800-323-
  Wolf
FAX: 708-913-6959
Offer:
  rigid laryngeal endoscopes
  stroboscopic light sources

video cameras

video recorders

video printers

video monitors

image management systems

Olympus   3.6 diameter

Fax PO to 1-800-833-1482   Attn. Lauren

01

KAT
Welch-Allen 3.5 $5950

3.4 diameter

Pentax   2.4 - 4.8

Fax PO to 1-914-365-0822 Attn: Kelly

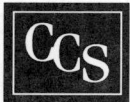

INDEX